FOREWORD

Jonathan Thomason has written a detailed and thought-provoking book. No surprise there - he is a man on a mission. He wants to tell the world about his work with ultrasound devices and the remarkable results he has seen in people he has attempted to cure over recent years. (Work medically confirmed by the Moffitt cancer centre)

His assertions won't please everyone. As he says, repeatedly, the Medical Establishment exist to supply a range of cures that they feel are 'tried and tested'. Unfortunately, as we all know, their current results are never one hundred per cent. Despite this, they seem reluctant to venture into new areas of treatment - unless they can be reassured with Papers and Research Results.

Meanwhile, the people who supply the Doctors, the massive pharmaceutical companies, are reluctant to veer off the path of best profits. As evidenced recently, with the complete refusal of such drug conglomerates to bother investing money in new antibiotics. As they say, there's not enough money in it for them! Unless the government steps in, antibiotics will become increasingly ineffective and even simple infections will become killers again.

Into this arena steps a new champion. Jonathan Thomason, hugely qualified in many fields, has arrived in health and treatment and is touting the ultrasound device as a cure-all for many of the killers of our age. It is a bold and brave campaign, and the future can only have two possible outcomes. One, the medical profession will take on what he says, try it out and prove it doesn't work. Or, the alternative, they will take it on, try it out and achieve massively better outcomes for their patients.

Either way, those suffering right now from horrible and deadly diseases, deserve nothing more than one simple thing - attention. Attention needs to be paid to the possibilities that JT is putting forward, and testing needs to be done, both in Britain and around the world. Ignoring this book; pretending the claims aren't happening; judging from known knowledge today without looking into Mr Thomason's experiences; will be nothing short of scandalous and will be a blot on the reputations of those called to the noble pursuit of healing and medicine.

Prof Mike Scantlebury April 2018

HIFU And Life

Highly intensity focused ultrasound and cancer

Dedication

My family members who have died as a result of cancer and diabetes. Also to all the medical geniuses who have shared their unique insights into human ageing and its attendant diseases.

Alison Cross MBE BA York 1978
Primarily to Dr. Polly MatZinger of the NI H
Ph.D. Chief, T-Cell Tolerance
Professor BB Argent Sheffield University BMet PhD DMet
The CEng FIMMM CPhys FinstP MRSC Emeritus
Professor H. Weiner Harvard Medical school
Professor Fossil Department of Geological Sciences
Michigan State College

Prologue

When a person has an infective illness, the virus or bacteria copies out the genome which gives it accommodation with the host, to share with other pathogens. When these 'pathogen leaders' get into a body cell or colonise a body tissue, they form a viral or bacterial rump.

The most important viral rump is cancer: which shares five enzymes with infective disease. Such rumps are both pressurised and under supported! All cancers employing the same single cell growth strategy used by all viruses.

This sort of cell division is used under very tight control by a growing embryo in its mother's womb. After birth, only the multi cellular cell division system is used by body cells. All viruses employ the single cell method-as does cancer.

Ultrasound at 150 W 40 kHz(HIUS. 2018 now 8W 1MHz from an ultrasound massage device) will selectively destroy the pressurised pathogen rumps. Clearing the diseases of age. The Americans started curing prostate cancer at one outpatient visit, using high intensity focused ultrasound in 2002.

Body cells are burned by ultrasound above 180 W/cm^2. But for the pressurised cancer cell, they experienced cell content boiling at only 90 W! So a HIUS causes explosive fragmentation our only of viruses and cancer cells. High Intensity Focused Ultrasound is a less efective form of High Intensity UltraSound - as explained later.

This will work for all cancers, heart disease, diabetes, mental health problems- MS, Alzheimer's, Parkinson's and schizophrenia, IBS, arthritis and the other diseases of age.

With no drug use or disfiguring surgery. Cancer has been cured 16 years ago. As has heart disease, diabetes, mental health problems and all infections.

Infectious bacteria are copied out by the B cells. Who mistake them for empathic structures. Until they start doing cell damage on day three. All bacterial replication there stops. The immune system replicates bacteria and give them a minimal cell wall.

Like viruses they demand and get extra blood supplies. So they are very vital-but cell structures are inflated and susceptible to HIUS. No body cell is over inflated-so HIUS is totally benign to innate cells.

All that drug companies are trying to keep this news out of the media! This book will tell you all about it! Live longer and prosper!

Medics talk as if cancer is random - or caused by a defective native genome! This is illogical rubbish. All 200 sorts of cancer out there share six common enzymes with other cancers and infective disease. They divide in a viral fashion.

I am an engineer, and this struck me as singular! It is not a random mutation! It is genome left behind from infective disease. We want six enzymes to form a cancer- so we get genome left behind by a person's infective history. Genome from many infections.

Those six enzymes make cancers and infective disease do their common stuff! They are about setting up secondary infection sites through the lymph system. The virus grows uncontrollably in a single cell fashion: I explain the significance of this point later in this book.

Never satisfied with its rate of growth, a cancer grows in the same way as viruses or amoeba do. But they have access to unlimited food and water. This trait is provided by endothelial growth factor. Don't the medics like all of their names!

In plain English (or American or translated into any human language) it means to make blood vessels grow. It is a demand for extra blood supplies.

This is a unique characteristic of body tissues and organs. But such demands should have been met by late adult state. They make requests for new blood vessels-usually only resulting from traumatic injury to body tissues.

So we can no more stop this trait than we can target cell growth: this latter approach has been tried against cancer with horrendous consequences for last 150 years.

All those six enzymes grouped together, should not occur in one specific locality. The immune system is sensitive to misplaced human enzymes and to foreign enzymes.

Not just to non native enzymes! Cancer falls under immune surveillance as its actions do not cause direct cell damage to body tissues. Growing fast is not in itself dangerous!

Giving a drip of interleukin two and four will produce an immune action against all such misplaced actions. But the drug companies are not interested in cures! Pills of the produced enzymes, would cure all cancers for 67p. They are so not intereted.

The medical world has no interest in producing human antibody pills to the common cancer enzymes, as this would cure all cancers with only one course of tablets.

All cancers misproduce six enzymes native to body Bio chemistry: but they are located in the wrong place for the wrong tissue type.

Over the decades in the last two centuries, medics have accidentally fallen across cures to cancer! The specific and general cancer cures. And then quickly shredded their notes. No money there!

There is no value in being such a total genius. Bio chemistry wants treatments-patients take until the day there patients die. There is no financial interest in curing cancer. 2 years of pills, then they die.

The medics realizing that such developments while immense for human life, would make no money. So with HIFU! None of us can see how anybody can make any money at a this technology.

Everybody gets to live. Medics have worse than zero interest in such technology. The Hippocratic oath dictates that everyone should work towards a cure. Financial self interest dictates otherwise.

The 1939 cancer act made work on a cancer cure criminal - treatments were the thing. Then cancer Research is the world's largest charity, that does not research High Intensity UltraSound - as it works.

The ultrasound has been used for 50 years to examine metallurgical forgings. Low power ultrasound has even been employed to image cancer tumours since the 1950s.

This is so curious! In response to low power ultrasound cancer cells to emit nuclear radiation. They do biological molecular nuclear fusion:
$H_2O+US->He+O+E^2+gwr$
gwr= gamma wave radiation. The exclusive province of nuclear reactions-are we are no source on nuclear fission.

Turning the power level up to destroy a cancer is an obvious idea! But it totally destroys the earning capacity of biochemistry and that drug companies. Destroying cancer is an obvious cancer cure.

Ultrasound is a physical cure! Evolved totally outside the biochemical and medical arenas. When I worked in metallurgical ultrasound I had not realized that this technology would have medical application. All the technology was developed for the examination of metals: well that's was job anyway!

We are not talking about a failing, fatal treatment for cancer. We are talking about a one session of ultrasound curing all body cancers. People will be jubilant They will be celebrating in the streets. Doctors and drug companies less so.

As you read this today drug companies are already filing for chapter Xi bankruptcy. Through my videos (JonThm on Youtube.com) text blogs ('Jons interests' on Blogger .Com) I have tried to ensure this information will reach everybody in the developed, and then undeveloped world.

The 3 medical professors at the Moffitt gave up on other medics using their ideas 2010. And retired. I have used their work majorly. I though of the initial idea anyway. Just didn't think it would work so well.

I told my old professor - but he still let medics medicate him to an agonising death. Clever guy. But not that clever. As Jesus said 'a profit is not recognised in their own town'.

Cancer affects all countries and people around the world. Though it is mostly a disease of the developed world. This is because there are more infectious diseases in the developed world; which spawn of the viral rumps which band together to form cancer.

Cancer is a post viral problem! So when we have an influx of viruses during engineer project-we see our local spike of cancers around the engineering plant. The early warning stations at the north of Scotland again the world centre for MS. It also is a post viral problem.

If we apply 8W 1MHz ultrasound to both sides of the chest, throat, nose and 20 seconds each side of the lower torso, we cure all infections, Stopping cancers, heart disease, mental health problems etc...

How the drug companies must hate me! But the cytokine idea, I outlined above is biochemical: it was produced with help from Harvard Medical School. You are probably quite confused-but I will give no more details. High Intensity UltraSound is better.

The ultrasound idea is a physical cure and so much easier to implement. Personal ultrasound devices generate the right frequency and power (150 W 40 kHz, now 8W 1MHz) to clear cancer from the body. Such devices are licensed for unsupervised human use. More details later!

As I mentioned above, I am an engineer. One of the four jobs I had, before my premature retirement for a car accident, was to work on metallurgical ultrasound.

I was back at Sheffield University doing a PH D into Chemical Engineering in 2001; making legal and medical history! After 30% brain damage you do not register for a higher degree. But there again, you do not have six e Books on Amazon Kindle. And I am working on my first full printed manuscripts on Lulu.com. I have 4 print on demand books with them.

I became aware they cancer was visible under low power ultrasound scans. I suggested using higher power ultrasound scans. I was meant to be doing a P_hD in Chemical Engineering at the time-and did not expect to the right! My supervisor was not happy - nobody is that bright.

The medics at the Moffitt cancer centre in Florida tried out high intensity ultrasound on prostate cancer. They <u>may</u> have thought of the idea totally independently-it was such an obvious idea. The cancer to emit gamma wave/X-ray radiation, suggested there was interesting science here!

It transpired the important thing was not the X-ray radiation. It was a massive production of heat in response to the ultrasound. This causes cell content boiling and the explosive fragmentation of the cancer cells.

This did cell damage to bystander body cells. That lie within the dendrite mesh! Cancer crushes into the gaps - hence the pain from growing cancers, The immune system sees the cell damage, the novel cell types locally and launches an immune action to clear the cancer cell throughout the body.

All primary and secondary cancer cells are history. We give the body the danger signal, to launch an immune assault - cancer does not usually produce. Local exploratory surgery MAY/may not give.

The 'be visible' I mentioned above, means converting ultrasound into nuclear radiation. Ideal for exposing photographic film kept in the dark. We already knew that X rays showed up the higher density cancer tissues. Gamma wave radiation is just a lower frequency X rays.

But now we have something altogether different! No external source of X rays. Cancer converted the higher frequency sound waves into nuclear radiation. This was actually the subject of my Chemical Engineering Ph.D..

Ultrasound causes the boiling off liquid water, by inducing physical molecular nuclear fusion at the 2kW 40kHz power range. My supervisor said he did not understand this system- he went off to lecture undergraduates and the steam cycle.

Steam in turbulent flow does molecular nuclear fusion. MNF is why steam engines generate so much energy. Producing Nuclear Fusion heat,

I was working on ultrasound doing molecular nuclear fusion. It used regular water with intermediate level ultrasound, and I already knew this heated up the water very rapidly.

Ultrasound is dangerous stuff! Metallurgical ultrasound can produce ultrasound burns on regular tissue - 180W 40kHz. But cancer cells experience cell content boiling even at low power levels of the ultrasound. 90W 40kHz.

It transpires the ultrasound also generated heat, as bubbles of gas pass through it -I learnt this during my metallurgical job in 1983(sic). We never did analyse those bubbles. We should have done. He and O gases. We smelt the ozone produced.

$$2H+O+TU+O_2 \rightarrow He+E^2+O_3+X\text{-rays}$$

They were composed of helium and oxygen gas. Read the last three sentences again! We transform regular water into helium and oxygen massive energy and X-ray radiation. Time to repeat that chemical equation! Such an important one.

$$H_2O+TU \rightarrow He+O+E+gwr/X\text{-ray}$$

This is modern alchemy. We transform two hydrogen atoms into one helium atom. This is nuclear fusion. This happens throughout nature. Where ever we have high pressure water or steam in turbulent flow. Which is why there is 5.125 parts per million helium in the air.

That is lost to space and replaced every day. Every biological organism on earth does biological molecular nuclear fusion. Professors of physics are not the right people to study this. It should be done by biologists.

Who are not so stupid as to fail to realise that global photosynthesis limits free carbon dioxide levels in the air to 2 parts per million. Extra carbon dioxide results in extra life on earth. It does not results in additional carbon dioxide in the air: that is nuclear power inspired biological fiction.

Molecular nuclear fusion produce a massive amount of heat! Nearly the energy equivalent of one hydrogen atom. The single radical oxygen ends up as ozone around the equipment. $O+O_2->O_3$

Life on earth is only possible due to the shielding affects of the earth's magnetic field and the ozone layer. Life can not exist in outer space - as far as we know! Without serious radiation shielding-the Apollo craft did not have. Even today we could not send men to the Moon and get them there alive.

They it would arrive DOA. The radiation field would have roasted them alive. So on the way to the Moon they will become blackened corpses. It is a point all American pride to believe the Apollo missions could have happened. Sorry. No they never did!

The water heats up very efficiently. We are talking about 10 seconds to boil a 2 pint flask of water. Outer space, you boil alive in 5 minutes.

We also get off He and O gases plus nuclear radiation and some heat! This is what low power ultrasound does to cancer cells. But cancer cells are pressurised.

Molecular nuclear fusion is exponential with pressure. So it does happen at room temperature. But if the water was pressurised, we can boil 1 litre in 10 seconds with 2kW ultrasound -data Sheffield University 2000. The 10,000,000°C of the sun is the product of all the nuclear fusion going on in the sun's Corona.

We even see nuclear fusion going on in the arctic seas! In deep sea currents at 3° C. Arctic fish give off gamma wave radiation and breathe out helium gas as their hearts and arteries do molecular nuclear fusion at -20° C.

But cancer cells demand extra blood supplies to grow - so end up overinflated and hard. As we pass low power ultrasound passes through body tissue, it wobbles and heats up by 16° C. Which produces nearly no nuclear radiation.

But body cells are more flaccid! And so we would expect to see little molecular nuclear fusion. All cancer cells are pressurised! So would expect to see exponentially more MNF.

Cell mitochondria and your blood stream in the heart and arteries do molecular nuclear fusion. So you biology gets heat from doing nuclear fusion. Your heart does it as it beats - as do the arteries, in time with your pulse. But cancer cells do a lot more!

In normal circumstances this gives them a vitality advantage. Cancer did not evolve expecting people to apply high intensity ultrasound to body tissue. Suddenly cancer does 10 times as much much heat generation as the cell can handle.

As your cells combine oxygen with carbohydrates, they do it! Time for another equation:
$C_m(H_2O)_n + (n-p)O_2 \rightarrow mCO_2 + pHe + (n-p)(H_2O + O_2) + E + X\text{-ray}$

This equation says combining oxygen with carbohydrates does a slow nuclear burn! It releases heat, X-ray radiation and produces carbon dioxide, oxygen and helium gases.

This is in the biology text books! But biologists are unaware that helium can only be produced by nuclear reactions. And we have no source of nuclear fission. So every second of the day and all bodies do nuclear fusion. Without us realizing!

So the human body naturally produces nuclear radiation from the physical molecular nuclear fusion in the blood stream, and the biochemical action of the mitochondria. So you are nuclear powered.

Biology gets 60% of its energy by doing nuclear fusion via the turbulent flow of high pressure water-or capitalised by a plant photo blasts or animal/and bacterial mitochondria.

The mitochondria combine oxygen with carbohydrates to get at the energy fuel cells need. Interestingly enough carbohydrates are produced from sunlight by photosynthesis. Which also produces nuclear radiation.

So both sides of the carbon cycle do nuclear fusion. Biology ensures there can be no builder of carbon in the atmosphere. Extra carbon results in extra life on earth.

So both halves of the carbon cycle do molecular nuclear fusion. Physics have never considered the nuclear fusion of hydrogen atoms could go off from compounds of hydrogen.

I atomic hydrogen doesn't really exist around the earth. Nature is four of molecular nuclear fusion.

Pressurise cancer cells do more of it naturally! So cancer would show up on passive X rays(sic)! Nobody considers this possibility, so never checked!

As cancer cells are pressurised, even 5W 40kHz ultrasound induces massive amounts of molecular nuclear fusion. Yes we get are significant amounts of nuclear radiation-so we can detect cancer by a photographic film.

It also produces loads and loads of heat! So ultrasound causes cancer cells to heat up by 60° C-when there cell is Bio chemically dead. Body cells <16ºC.

At 120° C the cancer cell boil and fragment explosively. This is noticed by the immune system, we clear the cancer cell type as undesirable, elsewhere in the body!

I know there have already explained this further on, so I'll leave you to enjoy that later! Nuclear Fusion in cancer cells - induced by high pressure sound. The beauty people use 8W 1MHz ultrasound. Medically licensed for safe home use.

In America, most personal bankruptcies are caused by medical costs - most defective cancer drug costs, The General Practitioner verified were defective medicine 2002, but carried on using.

Ultrasound below 180 Watts/cm^2 is benign to placid body cells. That pressurise cancer cells fragment above 90 W/cm^2.

The cancer cell being pressurised, is the unique defining characteristic of all cancers, that medicine has used to look for them successfully for two centuries. A simple ultrasound scan.

So if we apply ultrasound between 90 W and 180Watts we will selectively destroyed only cancer cells. Leaving regular body cells unharmed.

The Moffitt is desperately trying to produce a novel treatment option: which they can price accordingly! Their latest idea is High Intensity Focused Ultrasound, published physical science 20 years ago. Outside of patent protection. High Intensity UltraSound is more effective in removing secondaries anyway.

I talked about High Intensity Focused Ultrasound earlier in this book. It is the new hope of medicine to patent ultrasound. But it was science globally published by physics 20 years ago.

This instantly precludes it from any science patent. Your high school physics teacher can build a working kit - and blow all cancers away. No medical insurance needed. As I explain in this book, there is nothing magical about the ultrasound descriptions needed to destroy a cancer.

150W 40kHz was the first beauty ultrasound massage unit I used. Then 5W 1MHz, now 8W 1MHz. It really is that easy. You want power x frequency > 6 million W Hz. The beauty people use them to clear wrinkles, scars and lose weight.

The weight thing works, as the ultrasound blows away the fatty bacterial structure from the gut. The bacteria lays down the fatty sheath, to hide from the immune system.

We can safely remove this. But do 20 seconds first to the lower gut, then increase by 10 seconds a week. And you may get diarrhoea, take a week off, and resume 10 seconds less. Work up to 1 minute.

This will stop the 'trots' (Diarrhoea) we get when ill. It is caused by the immune system waking up to the bacterial rump. Which is why people can lose ½ a stone when ill. High Intensity UltraSound does this without the illness.

We also clear wrinkles and limb scaring - no potentially fatal surgery. So no 'body tuck' surgery is legal medicine any more. The Doctors struck off, for life.

It actually all is that simple. Once you stop trying to image cancer, and cause cancer cells to heat up and explode-it all seems so simple. My guess is that individual GPs found this out - and shredded their results - no money.

So the ultrasound so doesn't need to focus, the Moffitt is talking about concentrating the sound into a narrow beam. Very clever, but why? Cancer spreads out, we want a spreading out beam of ultrasound - like High Intensity UltraSound.

The power range required is very wide. The frequency is also not singular. I advocate 1MHz. This is a very effective frequency to boil off water at room pressure. 5W or 8W. Even 20W is safe, but really too rapid. Stick to 8W 1MHz - commercially available, and cheap.

If the water is pressurised we may only need 20 kHz. But I have not checked this! An 40 kHz will work just great. There is no price advantage in using 20 and 40 kHz. 2018 the state of the art for home beauty devices is 8W 1MHz. I started writing this book at 150W 40kHz, 1MHz 30 times cheaper to run.

Medicine became fascinated him pills - as they were not totally effective. But patenting the drug allowed massive prices. And the patients lives 4 times longer on drugs, than off. High Intensity UltraSound totally cues the cancer.

No Doctor or hospital involvement. If you High Intensity UltraSound your infections, you stop cancers, heart disease, mental health problems, asthma, IBS... The diseases of age.

You want ½ a minute each side of the chest, throat and nose. Plus 20 seconds each side of the lower torso. And then never need see a Doctor for a prescription. And no caners form, ever. Cancer not random or genetic - caused by a person's infective past.

Medical drugs will kill within four months to 10 years. When used its actually as advertised. Medicine does not want to do better! HIV is cleared by ½ a minute of HIUS to each side of the chest. Confirmed with an internet contact in New York.

Astra Zeneca became the world's richest country, by selling failing, inconvenient and ultimately fatal treatments. As cancer is now being cured, AZ has moved onto Statins.

According to Berkley, these add only 4 days to a heart patient's life - at massive expense. High Intensity

UltraSound for ½ a minute to the top left of the chest, and the kidneys.

Medics published about the kidneys 2012. The Hippocratic oath demands every heat Doctor read and confirmed this - using the High Intensity UltraSound device they bought to confirm the cancer cure 2002. Or ceased to be Doctors.

Not using High Intensity UltraSound since then has struck off all Doctors - included your General Practitioner. So you get back all medical costs since 2002. Your General Practitioner not s registered Doctor for 16 years.

All prescriptions invalid. Patients get all medical costs back, plus punitive damages - for an unlawful bankruptcy etc.. Medical practice for your GP, criminal for 16 years.

In this book I would describe in exact details how to cure cancer. This also works for diabetes and heart disease, mental health problems. For all the biggest killers of humanity.

No failing treatment. And the outright cure. How the drug companies must hate me! And all Doctors depend on prescription charges - now ALL illegal medicine. No Doctor can use.

When the medics in Florida first employed high intensity ultrasound on prostate cancer they produced the first cure to curing cancer in recorded history.

OK, it was my idea from Sheffield - but I had no idea it would work so well. On all 200 cancers. Thank you the 3 medical professors, who published the first 100 patient double blind trial on High Intensity UltraSound. I had called it HIU - though I was not happy with the name.

That did not involve around radiation to body tissues-and even there, so called cancer surgery and radio therapy has defective therapeutic outcomes. Secondary it usually killing the patient. There there is a mutilated body!

Using ultrasound, you increase the natural radiation produced by body cells, only in cancer cells. And you produce so much heat, the cancer cells boil away. All because mitochondria do Molecular Nuclear Fusion with ultrasound. Cancer cells, more Molecular Nuclear Fusion. And it transpires a fatal level of heat generation.

Ultrasound will selectively kill off cancer cells, while leaving body cells undamaged-explanation to follow! The drug companies have gone to great lengths to try and explain this cure away. They have no idea how it works - until they read this book.

My nursing friend has colon cancer, and read the chapter in my proof printed copy last night. He wrote down the details. I already cured him of heart disease.

And my step father of heart disease, colon cancer and diabetes type 2. Also my mother of type2 diabetes. That had killed 3 grandparents. My mother 'Diabetes is cured with a strict diet'. And a blast of High Intensity UltraSound!

Drug companies say HIUS only affects a few cancers! Never specifying their names or why they are especially susceptible. Because High Powered

UltraSound will CURE all 200 types of human cancers out there. In 1 minute - no drugs or Doctor.

Cancer is a post infection condition. So are all the diseases of age! I refer especially to coronary heart disease, mental health problems and diabetes. Coronary heart disease kills 12 million people around the world.

The British Coronary Foundation pays Doctors and nurses to use Statins. Now criminal medicine. All the Doctors and nurses shut down. Heart disease is now totally cured, 1 ½ minutes of High Intensity UltraSound; to the top left of the chest, and kidneys. ½ a minute externally to each area.

The biggest cause of global death - suicide. Biggest cause of suicide, medical fees - for prescribing defective medicine.

Diabetes only killed eight million. Including 3 of my own, non blood relatives. The reason cancer is susceptible to High Intensity UltraSound also makes these two conditions especially susceptible. A 1 session total cure - at home. No Doctor, drug company or hospital.

Applying HIFU to the coronary arteries and kidneys (explanation to follow) will cure coronary heart disease at one session. With no follow up drugs or surgery are appropriate. No Doctor involvement.

No requirement for heart transplants! All organs could potentially be repaired by using HIFU to clear away damaged cells. Without any requirements for organ transplantation.

There will be no requirement for liver transplantation. So no liver and heart swaps are required! They were only ever done as a have no better therapeutic outcome than heart transplants of donated organs, from a dead, and potentially infected person.

Leukaemia was treated with blood transfusion, to give them factor 7. Only trouble was, the patients got high levels of liver disease or HIV.

Now a blast of High Intensity UltraSound to the long bones, will clear the viral rump causing leukaemia. So curing the blood cancer. High Intensity UltraSound to the liver and kidneys, fully repairs these organs - removing infections. No transplants, total organ repair. No transplants.

Organ transplantation turns medics in to Dr. Frankenstein! Frankenstein was the Dr. involved in building the composite human that was the monster. Mary Shelley was intrigued that corpses sat up, on application of electric charges.

She would have been appalled that Doctors earn massive money, by transplanting organs from the dead. Next one, brain transplants. But High Intensity UltraSound will totally fix traumatic head injuries, and infections. No surgery.

Applying the ultrasound to the pancreas will cure diabetes: I had an e-mail from America saying this idea works! Sorry if I keep going on about this, but it is the practical demonstration that my ideas save lives.

The 8th biggest killer totally cured. No drugs. Type 2 diabetes ½ a minute of High Intensity UltraSound to the bottom right of the chest. No strict diet. Type 2, the full minute.

I have been steadily treating all her friends with arthritis. And there was a non-fatal condition, it is unpleasant. And he it is cured at one session of HIFU.

Asthma and IBS totally cured by local application of High Intensity UltraSound. ½ a minute each side of the chest for arthritis.

1 minute to the lower torso, for IBS and colon cancer.

My past

It was a fantastic IT career. It earned pocket falls of money. But it would not have helped humanity one iota: other than make cash point carts more convenient.

Aged 23 I was in one. the top 100 jobs of its type in the country. I was newly married. I knew nothing!

Now I work as a community video reporter, poet, over and folk lyricist and singer. Our next gig is to seeing an original song April 2013. By the time you read this, I will no doubt beyond to my 5th album.

That is not important! Your life is the most important thing in the universe! If I can't help them as human life, I will have succeeded. Show about the money!

Now I live at Salford quays. And three years ago was buzzing around in a BMW Mini. So I am not two harder! Wallpapers now he's on life. I owe it to whatever God you believe in.

I have put the first draft of this book out on Blogger, but a more extensive version will be available on Amazon books.

The latest version will be on Lulu. Am I trying to make money so this? No. I am trying to save life from the drug companies. Writing a book after my car accident was always impossible. I am trying to disprove that idea.

It will never get back our family members who have died from cancer and diabetes. Would that I had a time machine! We are all the same. We have lost special ones to the diseases of age.

Getting personal, they also lost myself to a car accident in 1988. But I'm still here. While you are alive you will not all down. Gold has use for all those!

I lost a wife, a career and a glittering future in IT through my car accident: the girl left me gently crying over her ruined futures. That's very poetic but not strictly true.

She went off their children will molecular. She never knew future. One without an attached crippled IT guy. I have a girlfriend after, who are fortunate died in a car accident.

She had a BA and a MBE = so called herself Bambe. She will be the hard act to follow. She had MS. Which is why I got interested in medicine= and got me in touch with Dr. MatZinger.

Polly MatZinger got me on my PhD: as I said further up, that made medical history. My training was not that of a medic. So I found non medical avenues of research.

It transpired these had great merit. I did not know about. I was just following up old job! By old boss had told me that ultrasound caused 'white finger'.

High power ultrasound (in the kilowatt range) damaged joint tissues. Di Jones was to retire and died of prostate cancer within six months.

While working in ultrasound, he was protected against cancer, heart disease, diabetes, arthritis, IBS, MS and the other diseases of age.

My first wife thought my story was over, and cut loose as catching the bus every day, day centre. I was looking after myself.

She left . I do mention fixing head injuries at the end of this book. It is possible to use HIUS (high intensity ultrasound) stave off all the diseases of age. Head and spinal injuries are just one element of human ageing.

I saw my wife again, she said I was with Alison. She had had 2 boys, one died in the first week. Presumably other children, by her new, Doctor husband. I wrote this book before I knew about him.

They has told her I had a new girl. But not that she had died. Her father and sister were Cambridge educated medics - so probably not the right girl. 25 years after we parted.

So maybe now I could fix me! My thanks go to professor Argent who contrived to get me back to Sheffield University. Through my research work I have now bought a High Intensity UltraSound device from China.

He died 3 years ago - from cancer. I told him the cure, but he stuck with the Doctors. And was dead in 18 months. I told him, he would be dead within 2 years.

In a year or two I will have to write a book about my journey's with my massage unit! And tell you how it all worked out. After my books on Nuclear Fusion and gold extraction.

A 34m meter bore hole to a magma chamber, located with ground sonar, will yield super heated water, with gold in. Vent the pressure, and extract the metal dust with a Dyson dry cleaner. Free power, and gold.

A ½m x 1cm steam plasma tube at 4 atmosphere will produce 2.4MW of heat: start up with the electronics from a fluorescent light. The plasma will self sustain.

A thermoelectric generator will produce 288kW of emission free heat: no CO_2 or NO/NO_2. The climate people have no given up on CO_2, justifying more hyper toxic uranium nuclear power. That needs 100 billion of annual insurance cover - per nuclear plant. None has - as not commercially available.

I went singing on stage, and that really helped my voice! Have been walking since 1989-but that has been a long journey back to near normal locomotion.

I was a struggling to be myself back at university, when a Dr. of immunology (Dr. MatZinger) got me on a P_hD into Chemical Engineering. Back at my previous university.

So I got a reference from America, to study science back at my English University. The staff there gave me some leeway to see what I would do. Prof Argent wanted me working with him - but he was not well enough.

I vindicated by old professor, by still demonstrating the intellect I had shown to the watching world, on my first degree. But now applied to Chemical Engineering and biology.

Chemical engineer was fair enough! That was covered on my master's degree. But biology I had last studied at my high school. Bolton School - such a good high school. Ralf Briton even taught me how to write. Never my thing.

I rapidly became aware that humans are a self replicating, Bio chemical engines. And engineering have taught me everything about how engines work.

Read all about by nuclear fusion ideas in 'Con-fusion' by Mike Scantlebury also on Lulu! I could give you the reference, but as your or read on the site just search by name. There is a guy of the same name in Belgium - but he does not write in English.

So so I wrote this book, I have written some more about how waterfalls do nuclear fusion. There are still working on that book for Lulu. But the early draft is out on Amazon Kindle.

It is now corrected, and Lulu are loving it. I told them to wait, to see how this book does. Writing is my therapy, and the courts gave me money for therapy. So I either holiday with it, or publish books. Which I have to write. And correct 27 times!

I am trying to demonstrate that everything relates to having access to nuclear fusion. Life he is amazingly special! Scientists say it is an accident of biochemistry. I tend to think that god had a hand here. Your beating heart, and cells give out X-rays, as they do Molecular Nuclear Fusion.

There is no reason that life could not arise in Computer Systems. Or may be I am biased-as my love affair with computers stretches back to the VIC 20 that I won from the Times Newspaper.

This was a computer, are produced before the Amiga; before Commodore, maker of the PET went bankrupt! As tends to be the way of high technology companies.

It was on my P$_h$D and I suggested using high powered ultrasound to restrict cancer growth. I then went off singing, writing and making videos - as you do!

That sort of thinking was novel to medics. Who promptly went off to check how it all worked. Or maybe they were looking anyway, and did not hear about it for 8 years.

What ever. Ultrasound worked a whole lot better than I could have envisaged. To have got a biological degree would have been a good idea - but then I would not have learned about ultrasound. My head would have been full of drug rubbish.

Fast forward to 2010, as my folk group was winding down. Then I read in a charity cancer magazine at Salford Royal Hospital that High Intensity Focused Ultrasound cures prostate cancer at one application.

Apply 8W 1MHz ultrasound from a massage device, for 1 minute to the gut over the penis. You may, or may not feel warming. My contacts said it worked. But nothing about warming.

This tackles the very nature of all cancers! I'll return to the subject often in this book. Utilising the science I learned in metallurgy, may save the lives of you and those you hold dearly.

Cancer cells must be pressurised in order to grow, in a viral fashion. High Intensity UltraSound causes such cells to pop. Leaving regular body cells undamaged.

With liver disease, the viral cells causing Hepatitis A/B/C all poop under High Intensity UltraSound. Even Hep C totally cleared in 1 minute - never any drugs. This medicine was known to ALL medics 2002 - you get back the last 16 years of liver cancer drug costs, your Doctor is struck off for life.

I can type, but for speed this is being dictated to my computer. Hopefully my proof readers will catch all the errors. And boy does it make errors! It transpires, I am my proof readers. This is my tenth pass through this book: never proof read your own writing.

Tonight I have added seven pages or even more to this manuscript. If I had had to type it that number would have been 4. Quick - but the errors!

And I make many errors: there are different ones to my dictation software. Which struggles with my nearly normal voice. Only speech therapists and voice recognition software can detect it is not normal.

The really crucial thing is to tell the world about the medical advances I have inadvertently learned about. OK, initiated and then returned to years later, to find they are now medically proved. And verified by every Doctor on Earth - or they were struck off 16 years ago.

Building on 'the danger model'-the incisive ideas of Dr. MatZinger at he NIH. I met her in Nottingham - clever lady. My P_hD got ended when Sheffield University found there has not totally focused on Chemical Engineering. Why? The best PhDs are produced by students with many, and varied interests.

My medical work, with input from leading medics around the world, made me aspire to be quite important. We are self replicating, mostly repairing, biochemical engines. And engines are my science.

I still never did got my P$_h$D though! That way I could have been paid to work on cancer. Sheffield University, never too late. Though the job offer has gone.

The problem would be, but being paid you put your head down and work on old ideas. I like new, radical thinking. My book publisher wants me to pay to be on a think tank - to get old ideas. Don't need them - in with the new and revolutionary.

You don't have the freedom to think outside the box with old ideas. But there again, you don't waste eight years of starvation on folk singing career. I like urban folk, but people are over it now. Now it is time to write crime thrillers - over to you prof Mike Scantlebury.

I would argue that song writing and singing was not a waste. I am getting internet from an X-factor TV producer about entering the show this year. But I have other uses for 2 years. Like writing an album. A classical, pop crossover.

And it didn't stop me thinking about cancer. The biggest waste of my time was trying about in my BMW. It did make getting around so easy - but boring.

It sure beats walking though. And don't tell me it keeps me fit. And keeps heart disease away. A buzz of High Intensity UltraSound does a lot better.

More effective - do it at home in 1 ½ minutes. As ever, my 8W 1MHz device. They last 3 years, but pay for themselves, as they cure you first infection: stopping cancers, heart disease, diabetes, mental health problems...

Such simple science - but a life changer. AS I mentioned above, cancers, heart disease, diabetes and metal health problems are now totally fixable.

The biggest cause of sudden death is suicide - caused by high Doctor bills: to prescribe defective, criminal drugs.

Apply the High Intensity UltraSound device for ½ a minute externally each side of the head, feel a lot better. And stop using that quack Doctor.

Who insists on prescribing defective, criminal cancer drugs, 16 years after they were ruled defective medicine.

Cancer cause

Medics have us believe that cancer is totally random! They fail to mention that all cancers share six enzymes in common with infectious viruses and even five with bacterial infections!

Work Cambridge University: who still insist on researching defective cancer drugs. Stop it - you are no longer registered Doctors.

Cancer is the result of an individual's infective past. This book will describe why that is so! It will then go on to describe the use of ultrasound to cure all cancers.

Biochemical companies were the richest in the world! But now the drugs are made in India and China. So the drug spend no longer goes to America. But American drug firms still source cancer drugs, in China etc..

Defective, illegal cancer drugs. Not legal to make and sell for 16 years. Doctors are not allowed to research or teach about them.

I maintain that a High Intensity UltraSound device is and already paid for, and validated major addition to the GP surgery.

Curing cancer, heart disease, diabetes, asthma, MS, IBS and mental health problems. These diseases of age are rise through an ageing population.

Curing them is an on-going process. My last chapter is on hearing the cells of age. This will stop the diseases of age and change human ageing. But it is a continuous process.

We should be in a constant state of body repair. Holding off the debilitating effects of ageing. We have the technology - and it is not 6 Million Dollar man implants, Rejuvenate your own body and brain.

Cancer leads to an agonising death in well under a decade. I presume the prognosis for heart disease and diabetes is much the same.

I know the life expectancy with MS is under 10 years:now totally fixable. My old girlfriend had this syndrome. It was she who first got me in touch with Dr. MatZinger.

The last time I saw her I was working on High Intensity UltraSound, but she died in a deliberately started house fire.

It was this seminar intellect they got me interested in cancer. The ultrasound stuff I knew from my job in metallurgical ultrasound. During my master's degree in to engineering.

I could have maybe got to Cambridge, but got my head full of old ideas. And not learn about ultrasound. Near miss!

Pathogen leaders

When a person is ill, their bodies are subject to the pathogen genome! An infection has the base 5 actions it needs to be a host specific infection.

This is very interesting issue to a biochemist. It means there are five common human antibodies to all human infections! The T cells make the antisense to novel genome. And attach IL-4. This human immune system enzyme gets a lot more mentions above!

My apply High Intensity UltraSound for 1 minute to a cancer - and the immune system makes the active antibody to clear the cancer from the body.

We repeat for 10 different cancers, and take blood samples. We select the 3 most important antibodies to cancer. Make pills of these enzymes, and get pills which cure all cancers for 67p. Neither drug companies or medics are interested, in actually curing any cancer.

HIV uses the IL-4 enzyme to get into white blood cells. It then hijacks this immune system oversight to churn out copies of itself. So the misusing the system that is there to make the antisense of the enzymes of infection, and cause the B cells to churn out copies.

If we apply HIUS for ½ a minute to each side of the chest, the AIDs cells boil and fragment. The body makes the active human antibody to clear HIV from the body. 100% effective, and it costs 13 UK pounds. For a total AIDs cure. Also works for Ebola.

I sent this idea to Liberia - end of Ebola outbreak 1. Outbreak 2 has also gone. Medics hope Ebola is AIDs II. Probably - totally fixable now.

There is no reason to get that involved! If we give a drip of IL-2&4, the immune system makes the human antibody. And the T cells loaded on the macrophages fraction. That is a function of IL-2. A quick buzz of High Intensity UltraSound, causes the body to make and action IL-2&4.

Some bright spark tried IL-4 on its own against cancer. But with no IL-2 it was never loaded on to the T cells, and then onto macrophages and actioned. The solitary antibody was cleared by the liver as so much junk! So close. But no hallelujah chorus.

If we give people with infections illness IL-2&4, their own immune system will make and action the active antibody. And cure the infection. We can take blood samples, get of the pathogen produced enzymes. And pills of the 5 common enzymes will cure all infective disease.

This is a natural, innate medicine. That your own body produces whenever you are ill and recovering. It can't be patented! The compatible drug makers should be making pills of this stuff by the ton. Nobody could ever undercut them.

American drug companies could never make a cent out of this idea. There will always be people who do not take pills, so the infections will continue to circulate the population.

Maybe at a reduced rate. But the drug companies in India and China could make a killing. By stopping infections killing. And we all get to live.

My interest in this biochemistry is that such a development would hold the promise of curing cancer and the diseases of age. Curing infections stops cancer, heart disease, diabetes, IBS etc. from the ever happening. This is an idea for them. But I am not a biochemist. Just your average smart engineer. We gave the medics joint replacements.

Mind you, now we can use High Intensity UltraSound, to totally fix joints and body tissues, and avoid the need for all surgery. We can even fix the brain, or traumatic injuries and strokes.

I have a master's degree in engineering. After and during my degree, I worked on ultrasound. This provides a simple physical cure to the diseases of age. That is what this book is all about.

Biochemistry and ultrasonics will be in competition. Biochemistry has a massive head start. And medics do not understand ultrasound: I am not sure that any body does. The box I have been written.

I was staggered to see there are three books about HIFU. Which is less effective than High Intensity UltraSound. But published physical science 20 years ago: so out of all science patents.

The acronym 'High intensity Focused Ultrasound' was the only medically adopted in 2011, for an old physics idea. Already there are people writing, who claim to understand it.

And fairly sure they're not 0,000 words to say about it. This is my contribution. From an ultrasound expert. Who actually understands it - another 30,000 words +.

As mentioned elsewhere in this book, I was doing a P_hD into Chemical Engineering in 2000: with my head injury and decade long rehabilitation this actually made a world record! But it went totally unnoticed. To did a higher degree with your injuries - not possible!

I have to remind myself every week, that I should not be alive. I should not be making a positive contribution to life. I suggested the use of high powered ultrasonics to restrict cancer growth.

It works better than I ever thought possible. So I have as much right as anybody to talk about it. The drug companies are trying to restrict knowledge of this development. Sorry. Life is rather more important than drug company incomes.

The common activities done by pathogens includes things like setting up secondary infection sites and denuding the host immune system of vitality.

Bacteria trick the B cells into thinking they are empathic organisms! So the immune system cells copy the bacterial genome, and even give it a minimal cell wall.

Bacteria can only replicate with the help of a multi cellular body! In the seas bacteria do replicate. But these tricks do not work in a multi cellular body. The inactive immune system is not too careful about replicating bacteria.

Its criteria is 'no local cell damage going on nearby'. If not, the bacterial must be harmless. And beneficial to life. It is empathic! The immune system links everything to cell damage. Cancer replicates as a virus, within mankind, but it cell damage is not noticed.

As I mentioned elsewhere viruses and bacteria divided using the single cell methods - as taught to me by professor Fossil. He thought I was a radical intellect. I am a creative thinker.

The most importantly, I have a master's degree in engineering. Not biochemistry of biology. So my ideas were different than medics!

Cancer can't divide using the multi cellular stem cells: as a check to see if there cells are is appropriate are needed. Viruses and cancer sidestepped this check by dividing like amoeba. Like most life on the planet.

They are more complicated than bacteria. And they only exist in the body with high levels of cell necrosis- not seen by the clustering dendrites: the dendrites form the supporting dendrite mesh in the body.

They monitor cell replication. Cancer cells must avoid their attention. So engulf all tumour cell death, before it is seen by the clustering dendrites of the immune system. The body's house keepers.

All necrosis within the cancer tumour is engulfed by surrounding cancer cells. So the dendrites never see any loose DNA/RNA. Exploratory cancer surgery does cell damage local to the cancer.

And half the time this cures the cancer. High Intensity UltraSound is 100% effective - as it makes the cancer cells pop. Spraying RNA into the blood stream.

The cancer cell also excrete IL-10 which turns down this immune action. During exploratory surgery squeezing the cancer tumour with forceps would release massive amounts of loose DNA. DNA is a potent immune system danger signal!

Small pox makes IL-10, but was overcome, as we gave vaccinations of cow pox, A non fatal virus in people. That pre-arms the immune system against pox viruses.

If we give cows with foot and mouth disease 2 minutes of High Intensity UltraSound to either side of their chest, they get totally better. And can't catch F&M for 40 years.

Again I must remind myself that I'm dealing with High Intensity UltraSound, and High Intensity Focused Ultrasound: which avoids all need for drug use or surgery.

Ultrasound causes cell damage around the cancer from outside the body. I will explain more about this below. I wrote this book over 16 years, and am always fascinated to read my thoughts from years ago.

Naked DNA/RNA is removed from the body, as a matter of course. After three days the infection has taken root, and the bacterial actions cause cell damage to body cells. After three days viruses also do this! This gives the pathogen a three day lead on the immune system.

Hide all cell damage for 3 days, to get established. And maybe kill the patient.

Cancer divides in a single cell way, and does no damage to body cells -naturally. We do not have to play by the rules of nature. Viruses and bacteria, and so cancer do no noticed cell damage.

As Dr. MatZinger observed with Dr. Mel Cohn, cell damage is a crucial factor to let tumours and cancers grow, with no immune action.

He does not get a name check or credit earlier in this book, but Dr. MatZinger has exchanged emails and formed this seminal idea, of cancer danger masking as a result.

Mel Cohn never even answered to my initial greeting! I have no doubt he is the seminar intellect. He is busy in California! We get back to the issue, Doctors are only interested in drug ideas.

I have been to California 3 times recently. And if I was living in California I might not be too bothered to exchange emails with a scientist, out to their field. The greatest advances in science have been made for scientists working out of their field.

Viruses are a lot more complicated than bacteria! They copy their own genome so are not strictly parasite like bacteria. Medics have protested for 40 years that fungal antibiotics should not work on human viruses. Yet doctors still prescribe them.

Fungal antibiotics should not work on human infections of any type! They actually stimulate the human immune system, so the antigen presenting centres churn out the active human antibodies, to the cell causing cell damage, inducing a full, normal immune action to any viral or bacterial pathogen.

They have no direct action. The only catch is, the human infection must be totally cleared well we are still taking fungal antibodies.

Otherwise we engage the allergic response, and become resistant to that fungal antibiotic. We can use low strength antibiotics, to turn off this allergic action - when well.

I have already written by section below on the allergic response: giving IL-2&4 engages this system to novel genome in the body. So we can use it to clear HIV, SARs, Ebola, diabetes, cancer and heart disease.

But the allergic response is undone the next time that allergic substance is in the blood stream with no cell damage. Cancer enters through infective disease and lungs. So each instance of cancer will require a new set of human antibody pills.

But, as I have mentioned, there are 6 antibodies common to all cancers etc..

We do not give interleukin 2&4 all the time. We take blood samples, and get out be much shorter human antibodies. There are five common antibodies to all infection.

But Doctors will not play along. So we give a quick buzz of High Intensity UltraSound (½ a minute each side of the chest …) and cure all infections, stopping all cancers etc..

If we give pills that are the active human antibody to stop single cell division, we stop cancer and infectious disease. We also stop live childbirth! So they are an on demand contraceptive. That does not leave a lasting immune memory - because the allergic response is routinely deleted. Evolution had thought, to not make all women infertile after 1 infection.

Such pills would have a constant demand. The drugs are produced naturally, but our only obtained by medics using artificial stimulation. When there they can be patented I do not know.

Certainly every person getting better from an infection produces these antibodies naturally. But they have never been identified or isolated in human history. Again, Bio chemistry is in tension with HIFU.

All pathogens share out strips of their genome-I term pathogen leaders. These are liberated into the bloodstream of strips of RNA, when there have been gobbled up by other pathogens but also cessated cells!

This was such a useful concept, I devised the name 'pathogen leader' in 2000. I was reading a copy of nature immunology six months later, and the name was already in use in the medical establishment!

It is quite possible the name predated my ideas. As it is followed American naming conventions. I am English. So what the hell happened there!

As viruses and bacteria found out how make a cell cessate even with available telomere. So the bulk of cessated cells, unless you live in an area of frequent famines, are pathogen in nature.

It is so useful for viruses to turn a body cell into a virus replicating robot. Ceasing biological activity, and just copping out the altered viral genome.

Every cell bud off the stem cells, have 50 divisions before the cell cessates, they are not cleared routinely by the macrophages and replaced by new cells.

The macrophages are persuaded to leave their cessated cells alone until the next famine. They act as an on body food store.

They also give a ready home to invading viruses and there fragments, pre and full cancer clusters. In modern society they serve no real scientists to humans. Through evolutionary history they were a massive advantage from hunter gatherers to early farmers.

In the days of the convenience store, they serve no human need. We are best without them. An infection often leads to their partial removal - and weight loss.

Not so much use now, to the supermarket generation! We neither need nor want such cells about. I do return to this toxic cause the end of this book. Right now it is the final chapter, but I am still writing the book. So who knows!

This trick resulted in a viral SARs becoming bacterial SARs. See my chapter on HIV below! This trait of infections to share genome is why pathogen enzymes show up in all infections!

Cancer is not random; it is built like LEGO® from your infective past. The diseases of age are all the result of pathogen leaders left behind from full infections.

This predicts that the cure to infections like the common cold will be the cure to cancer. So it has transpired to be!

½ a minute to each side of the chest, throat, nose and 20 seconds each side of the lower torso clears all viral and bacterial infections. At home with your HIUS device. Or at great cost, at he GPs using their HIUS device.

Never any fungal antibiotic pills prescription. Now succeeded, inferior, criminal medicine.

Bacteria and viruses are life on earth - just like us! We exploit other life forms for food -plus labour, shelter and warm.

So pathogens are just acting in exactly the same way. They earn their living by exploiting other life forms. They are not evil.

No more than we are! I personally am nice - I think. My enemies will disagree. They can write their own books. I just will not be reading them.

My contribution

I am not a medic. I have a master's degree in engineering. And following a serious car accident I had term to divert to my hobbies: singing, making videos, creative writing, curing MS and fixing me! I suffered 30% brain damage in the car accident.

It took me 8 years to be back on a P_hD - making medical history. Heaven is all very nice, but I was sent back to do stuff on Earth. I was not ready to die. That choice was never given me.

My first wife left in 1993. Thinking I would never make a positive contribution to life. Or a massive amounts of money.

What she's doing I don't really care: OK. Found out it was a lot of present knowledge nursing. Helping cancer patients to die in agony. My second wife, who I never officially married, died in a house fire 2004.

Divorce, the grieving is over in two years. Death of a partner takes a decade and for ever! Life now is getting very busy. I am singing on stage. Writing folk lyrics.

I am even though of a BBC media city gospel choir. They keep threatening to make me very busy. And doing the X-factor for ITV - watch this space.

When I get time allowed to practice my breathing for a few minutes: otherwise I would die! Then I do my job as a community video reporter. Now I also manage to be a free poet! That is how I got song writing.

When I'm through working on this book I have to help with major fiction writing for Mike Scantlebury.

I am the technical consultant for his book on nuclear fusion. I need to get back to the manuscript and add some jokes.

My book publisher is very impressed about my book on waterfalls doing Nuclear Fusion - as the water molecules collide, they produce He and O gases, X-rays and massive free, non toxic heat. With no Fossil Fuels burn.

As I also write radio comedy programmes. Not many today, as my breathing takes priority! And my singing, video making, doing poetry...

In 2000 my old professor got me to return to university. Arguing that before my car accident I had written the single most incisive essay ever penned by an undergraduate. He died 2015.

It concerned the failure by nuclear power to take account of the costs of decommissioning all its plants (and reprocessing its toxic waste). Decommissioning is actually dearer than building a nuclear plant.

This argument still applies today! The cost of decommissioning the plants and reprocessing the fuel is 10 times greater than generating power. EDF have stored the used fission rods in water tanks, to hand the cost of reprocessing the fuel on to future generations.

They have also extended the working lives of the aged nuclear plants beyond their design life. I used to work in heavy engineering. You don't do that sort of trick!

As technology advances, things get cheaper. And more reliable. Aged engineering plants breaks down! And cost a lot to maintain in working order. Nuclear plants are designed to wear out after 25 years. Don't try and extend their working lives - or you will get another Chernobyl/Fukishima/3 Mile Island/Windscale.

The Labour party sold British nuclear power off to EDF for €14,000,000,000. Probably the life extension of the nuclear plants was written in to the deal.

As of today only Sizewell B should be operating. Fukishima demonstrates that he did nuclear plants are accidents waiting to happen. Even if you are the most technologically advanced race on earth.

A new Hinkley C, would require annual insurance cover of 100 billion - not available. Fukishima has for ever bankrupted Japan.

Japan and Germany have renounced nuclear power. We allowed the French to operate 18 nuclear plants in the UK - now sold off to China, who hate the UK. 17 of which are beyond their design lives.

We need to AN INDEPENDANT plant power analyst and danger money! Nuclear power is probably going to kill us all very soon.

This is a unique element to the cost of producing nuclear power. My essay was two years before Chernobyl demonstrated the other unique failure of nuclear power.

It kills on a continental scale. It is the least green industry that will ever exist. Even before Global Warming, man-made Climate Change or Global don't make me laugh.

Plants take in carbon dioxide to grow. In the Jurassic age there were no fossil fuels, but 65% more life on earth.

So present photosynthesis is living in a time of denuded life. As we burn the fossil fuels we restore Jurassic Life to the active environment. Burning carbon fuels increases life. Nuclear power kills it. Anyway back to High Intensity Focused Ultrasound AND High Intensity UltraSound.!

My thoughts on safe clean nuclear fusion is contained in the novel 'Con-fusion' by Mike Scantlebury. That is not what this book is about!

Mike 'employed' me as a the nuclear technical consultant. And dedicated the book to me. When I finished with this book.

I intend to do more work on his volume. As he does not have the sick sense of humour I you have got! Life and death happens. It is part of life, and death.

There are no checks in this book - or very few! As I find nothing about cancer remotely funny. I seem to remember have already said this. Just to reiterate the point.

2001 my then girlfriend got me to watch a Horizon BBC TV show on the seminal work by Dr. Polly MatZinger of the NI H.

All these years later, her work has led directly to this book. Her mentor died before she had had the bravery to dedicate a novel to him.

You will notice that I have mentioned her repeatedly an even dedicated this for to her. Her work is that important, and with Amazon you can ensure you say the important things.

Her great contribution to science, is to find out the lack of substantive cell damage done to body cells by cancer.

The work on ultrasound I only suggested as a novel treatment. I have yet got to make the singular contribution that she he has done.

She always said that my gift to the future was my work on nuclear fusion: I really must get around to working on my Mike's book!

Cancer is the uncontrolled growth of non-differentiated cells. I suggested while on a PH D into chemical and process engineering that we should try ultrasound to restrict cancer growth.

Polley was intrigued by my systems ideas. This was just the stuff that was taught to me. My master's was all about applying other people ideas, in new areas.

Professor Bernard Argent always encouraged me to apply ideas from one area into another tenuously connected science.

One of the last times I saw him he congratulated me on my work in biology. I think he was being sarcastic as at the time I was on my Ph.D. into Chemical Engineering.

My degree in was in systems work, and the biggest system on this planet is the natural weather. For medicine, the biggest system was cancer growth.

So all these years on and still doing Systems Engineering! The biology was in large part due to the import of information from Dr. MatZinger.

Augmented by my excessive coffee consumption at the time! I have sleep scheduled for a week on Tuesday.

We are talking major coffee consumption here. The world's most important drug. No drug firm involved.

I have worked in metallurgical ultrasound, and was aware that medics used a lower power ultrasound. This I fact was singular!

Cancer tumours were opaque to ultrasound - and they gave out X-rays. I got on with trying to do my P_hD though.

And left medics to research this area. Physicist could have helped the medics here. And told them they have stumbled on a nuclear reaction without any radioactive isotopes.

Prof Agent called this Molecular Nuclear Fusion. It goes on in all life on Earth - and physical systems with high pressure water, or steam in turbulent flow.

Medical ultrasound produces gamma wave radiation/X-rays, when striking a cancer etc. cell. Animal biology does this in areas on earth.

Plants also do Molecular Nuclear Fusion. Physicists need the help of biological or medical students to study this area.

Life does nuclear fusion from water. No plutonium. No uranium, plutonium or strontium involved. Nuclear guys. Get over it. Life does nuclear fusion from water.

In 2002 the Moffitt cancer centre did not employ the higher power ultrasound I had recommended. They used high intensity focused ultrasound.

Which to you and me is a less effective High Intensity UltraSound! I guess I should explain a bit more at this stage.

The whole purpose of this book is to describe how HIFU does not image cancer; it is of one appointment cure to all cancers and the other diseases of age out there! Get yourself a drink, ensure you have clean underwear on and here we go!

High Intensity Focused Ultrasound

When I first wrote an article about this, I did not read the article on High Intensity Focused Ultrasound! Because you can't focus sound with a glass lens.

You can angle it around corners, using a massive structures. The body is not a massive structure - unless you eat a lot of chocolate bars!

You can produce coherent ultrasound - as a laser is coherent, focused light

I should have remembered during World War II they erected parabolic listening reflectors, to concentrate the noise of an aircraft engine to give early warning of the approach of aircraft.

A precursor to, and less effective than radar - which uses microwave radiation in place of sound.

The devices were never used as radar was 100 times more effective. In the same way that a parabola can concentrate sound waves, emitting ultrasound on a guide tube produces, a slowly diverging cone of acoustic sound!

A laser beam of sound. This will pass directly through the body. Even I do not know it all! I had some book work to do. About 6 months of work.

I thought a bit more about focusing sound. You can't focus the ultrasound, but you can concentrate it! If you emit ultrasound down a closed end cylinder it will emerge as a diverging cone of acoustic energy. Maybe this is 'focused' - just call me a pedant.

We emit coherent sound from crystals. In the same way stimulation of crystals produces coherent light.

It certainly is a lot more concentrated than the sound diverging from a loudspeaker. In use will cut through metal. This is why physics got interested 1988.

But the same light not focused we'll just illuminate the metal structure. Concentrating the ultrasound into a small beam allows us to do magic.

Lasers are the greatest technological advance of the early 20th century. They allow CD/DVD/Blue ray drives to work.

And I have got five in my house! Only one set of ears. I am corresponding with God over this design problem. Concentrated ultrasound destroys cancer cells. But so does 8W 1MHz ultrasound, from an acoustic emitter, in HIUS.

Standing in front of a rock band, their speaker may have some small effect, making you and drinks wobble. But it will send you prematurely deaf! High Intensity UltraSound can fix your hearing.

Deafness is what medics call an insurmountable, unwarranted side effect. This is why rock music curing cancer never made it out to the starting gate.

A quick search of the intimate uncovers the fact that ultrasound is toxic to body cells at moderate power levels - 180 W/cm^2. That is a brisk walk up the hill, and standing on one foot for 10 seconds! Not really high intensity. No more than it is really focused!

I am used to metallurgical ultrasound. Where are we are dealing typically at 2 kW. Now that is high powered. The biohazard gear you are advised to wear to wear is considerable! To protect medical problems like white finger. I knew this in 1983.

As mentioned elsewhere my old boss retired and died of pancreatic cancer. This is a common problem! People retire, and six months later are dead.

Manual workers are exposed to ultrasound through life. Driving a car exposes a person to intermittent moderate level X-ray radiation. This obviously requires me to write the book. Work may stop some cancers. Retirement kills.

Sheffield University have all the occupational health data on record. An engineering lecturer even reminded me about the occupational health effect of retirement.

And until you know about HIUS it makes no sense. My head was full of nuclear fusion. Which I can assure you hurts. Your body cells and bloodstream both do low level biological Molecular Nuclear Fusion.

At a lower level than cancers does naturally. We increase the level of MNF by applying ultrasound at power levels not detrimental to body cells. Which will cause cancer cells etc., to pop.

My P_hD got ended as I got interested in cancer and biological stuff. Yet Cambridge and Harvard did not fall over themselves to get me to do a biological Ph.D.. My ideas were too far ahead of air time. And that is what this book is all about!

University science is 20 years away from application. The work on lasers and CDs was done in their mid sixties. Conventional CD players came in the eighties!

HIUS will totally alter medical comprehension and teaching in universities. Hence Harvard in Cambridge are a bit reluctant to engage.

I first learned about the miraculous nature of ultrasound while working in non destructive testing at Inco. Here we were using ultrasound in the kilowatt power range to examine metal forgings. Special protective clothing had to be worn.

No scientist has ever commented that steal forging cracks release nuclear radiation in response to ultrasound! We get off X-ray radiation and produce macroscopic bubbles of He and O gases, from the ultrasound fluid: water and fat! Peter Cutler showed me this in 1982. I thought it was curious!

Back on my P_hD in 2000 and the cold fusion work was out. This used a combination of radio and sound waves to turn water into helium and oxygen gases, with loads of heat, and a little gamma wave/X-ray radiation: this was Molecular Nuclear Fusion.

I thought up the idea. But Professor Bernard Argent modified the name to be less biological and more physical: molecular (nuclear) fusion. He realised that at the time I was getting increasingly into biology.

Harvard has also published a document on the release of gamma wave/X-ray radiation by all life. This can only be produced by nuclear reactions! And the body avoids toxic nuclear fission! Any cell damage by nuclear fusion is cleared routinely.

In animals we get a burst of biological MNF in the heart and arteries as the heart beats. The emission of gamma wave radiation is on medical records. Without any explanation. Biologists being unaware they have just proved animal life does nuclear fusion from water.

Green crops in light produce helium, free radical oxygen, heat and X-ray/gamma wave radiation. So all life on earth is in part supported by the energy release from biological Molecular Nuclear Fusion.

This allows green crops to expose photographic film in a light tight envelope, exposing it instantly! I learned about this in 1978. Thank you Dr. Shaw at Bolton School! He never explained why. Because nobody knew why then.

But cancer is more vital than body cells! So it does more MNF than regular body cells. From my metallurgical work I knew that ultrasound causes rapid boiling of water.

It did physical MNF. If you expose cancer to High Intensity Focused Ultrasound/High Intensity UltraSound , the cancer infected cells do toxic levels of MNF! Causing cancer etc., cells to boil off. Inducing an immune action to clear the distinct cancer type.

The cancer cells explode as they are exposed to moderate power levels of ultrasound. I am pretty sure that cancer cell fragments at 120° C. Like all cells, they are dead at 60° C.

The fragmentation is so explosive we destroy bystander body cells. And this produces the four immune action against cancer.

That cancer does not provoke an immune, cleansing action, naturally. Now the induced immune action clears cancer cells throughout the body.

Primary and secondary cancer clusters history. This is so useful! We can destroying the bulk of primary cancer cells, in the wake, the immune system will clear the rest.

Attending regular rock concerts has not taken off as an alternative protection against cancer! Rock artists probably have lower cancer rates, when performing.

All this sound energy, might stop, or you ended up with painful, immobile joints - white finger in the rock world. This was a subtle hint that there was important science I should investigate. Instead I studied metallurgy, and got my master's degree.

I liked my rock music as much as the next man. 2014 I performed with my folk group, OldSorts on theatre stages through Salford. It is essential to think creatively, to vent your creative muse in artistic pursuits. I have drawn and painted. Today I singer and write folk lyrics.

In 1986 I moved to London to work in Lloyd's Back in IT. Then I nearly died in a car accident. So I got divorced. And got together with another girl. And embarked on a P_hD.. Then I learned to sing. All through these years Polly Matzinger get me focused on cancer.

I still sing as a hobby - X-factor - who knows! I like my creative writing and my singing. I could have made a useful career out of either perhaps. Instead I did science.

Unwittingly in 2001 I heard about ultrasound and the public health date; so I sent my medical contacts my ideas about ultrasound.

It then required medics to do some work. I read about this work in a cancer charity magazine while at hospital for a routine appointment 2010.

You can imagine how pleased I was t read that ultrasound did not just treat cancer - as I had suggested. Since 2002 the Moffitt cancer centre has been curing prostate cancer at one appointment using High Intensity UltraSound/High Intensity Focused Ultrasound .

They did not realise they have the answer to all body cancers! Working and it could be routinely used in every consulting rooms.

Ultrasound targets the innate nature of cancer - that is overinflated and under supported. Medicine has been trying to locate this unique angle of attack for two millennia. A Roman emperor's wife died from 'a growth'.

The Roman emperors wife died from a malignant growth in the first century of the Christian calendar. Cancer has been with us ever since ancestors diverged from the reptilian line.

As mentioned elsewhere, reptiles do not get cancer. As Brigitte Bardot mention, being pregnant is like having cancer. A foreign growth taking over your body, and growing like mad.

She was so correct! She had a massive medical insight. A live embryo has DNA that is half from the father. So is foreign to the mother.

The placenta does loads of stuff to damp down the immune system. This makes pregnancy a peak time for bad viruses and cancer to develop in a mother.

If we give interleukin two and four to a person with an infection, will get the human antibodies. To infections. The top six antibodies will cure all infections and cancers, and also acts as an on demand contraceptive.

This is why an infection often leads to a mother miscarrying. It provides the missing cell damage signal. The local antigen presenting centres, of the immune system make the human antibodies, but also interleukin 10 to damp down the immune system away from the infection.

The human antibody with no interleukin 10 will render the mother selectively infertile, as she takes the pills. One month after stopping the pills she can become pregnant again.

Ultrasound is totally amazing . I was staggered. They had devised a power range of ultrasound in Florida that cures prostate cancer at one appointment. This exploits the over inflated and under supported nature of all cancers. HIUS must cure all cancer.

Savour that thought for a moment! No expensive ultimately failing biochemical treatment. A 1 appointment total cure to all body and brain cancers. The drug companies are going to is so upset about this. They needn't be.

Drug companies will move on to offering biochemical six months regular treatments, to prevent the diseases of ageing. Your own High Intensity UltraSound device is a cheaper way of stopping ageing. But we want the Doctor.

By clearing cessated and genome altered cells out of the body! They will keep people healthy! Which is what we have been paying for anyway. Drug just had slowed down our descent to death. And persuaded us it was the same thing!

Regular High Intensity UltraSound use stops ageing, and the diseases of age.

The other diseases of age share these characteristic: they have cells are both are overinflated and under supported.

Ultrasound will cure them all! Suddenly my singing original songs on stage did not seem that important. Ultrasound does not just cure cancer: it cures heart disease, diabetes, IBS, arthritis and the other diseases of age.

If used on a routine basis it will prevent these diseases occurring. By curing all infectious diseases. This future has just been changed.

Diabetes is one such disease. That drug companies are targeting as a major income stream-as cancer is cured!

They thought this would be over the next 50 years. They could hardly believe their eyes when the Moffitt cancer centre started curing prostate cancer at one appointment of HIUS in 2002.

This work was transferred directly across to pancreatic and other cancers. A disease that has influenced life and lead to my work on ultrasound.

Pancreatic cancer is a bed fellow of diabetes. For biology in both cases demonstrate the presence of hardened cells. These are a viral rumps. The structures causing cancers, heart disease, mental health problems and diabetes.

I must give tribute here to and an unnamed medic, who published an article in 2008 saying that the heart disease was characterised by hardened bacterial structures on the coronary arteries. This was when the main medical ideas, caused my thinking about viral and bacterial rumps.

So the idea did not come out of the air! It was based on existing published medicine. This was important in my ideas about HIUS. I was away singing on stage

2003 until the present day. Medics did the legwork and formed the occupational date work. Sheffield University completed the idea on viral rumps.

My degree was all about systems! How changing one area of men in the dark, had unexpected results. Medics knew that cancer cells were overinflated and hard: but they were always making too much money from biochemistry.

As an engineer, I found this very interesting! It related to the work I was doing on ultrasound and nuclear fusion. Without the Moffitt cancer centre trying it all, I wouldn't have got nowhere. All the elements of HIUS were out there. Published in scientific journals!

But biology is do not read physics science journals. And engineers do not read biological science journals. I only engage with biology at the urging of Dr. Polly MatZinger. She was impressed by my physical knowledge, than as water froze, it expanded!

So global warming - had it ever happened, would the melted the polar ice and and lowered sea levels. My systems work highlighted the importance of global photosynthesis.

The fossil fuels formed 65 million years ago. At the end of the Jurassic age. When the 85% more life on earth, and sea levels were 60 metres lower.

This system drives life on land and in the seas. Burning the fossil fuels resurrects ensured life. Photosynthesis ensures the trace of carbon dioxide left in the air at the end of the day has remained static for 200 years. At just 2 parts per million/ 200 ppm - biologically impossible, with global photosynthesis.

The carbon dioxide level can only rise in a natural ice age, or above the Arctic ice caps, in winter. There is no weather effect!

We have natural ice ages with higher levels of CO2. Sea levels go down as the ice sheets grow. So we are at a period of natural fixed sea levels.

This will fall as life on earth over the land and in the seas increases. Biology teaches that the limit to global life is circulating organic carbon. Man made climate change is spurious fiction from the diseased pens of nuclear power.

Man is restoring natural life to the Earth. The Fossil Fuels are life locked away.

Since when did you take biological advice from individuals totally ignorant about photosynthesis: and take it from a power physics professors-with large research contracts to nuclear power.

This was why I was never awarded a P_hD. for pointing out that man made global warming was biologically impossible. Because photosynthesis converts additional carbon dioxide <u>back</u> into active biology.

But my thoughts about Molecular Nuclear Fusion lead on to my ideas about ultrasound. Which went on to a one appointment cure to all diseases of age. With MS, we need to spread out the HIFU over 10 sections-as we apply the ultrasound to the head.

This is wrong, in 2013 I cured a man of MS, using ½ a minute of High Intensity UltraSound to each side of the head, just once. The man stopped after 20 seconds.

For too long biochemistry has a ring fenced cancer, in the same way physics has a ring fenced nuclear fusion: saying 'this area is ours, keep out'.

All living organisms on earth give out X-ray radiation and produce helium gas. Plus free radical oxygen and energy.

Any physics professor would tell you these are symptomatic of nuclear fusion. They did not consider biological molecular nuclear fusion was a possibility.

Chemists knew about the emission of nuclear radiation from chemical reactions from the 1970s. They never completed the circuit and investigated chemical Molecular Nuclear Fusion.

I am a post graduate metallurgist. Specializing in radioactivity. Even on my P_hD in 2000 it took another P_hD student to tell me 'steam engines form helium' for me to even contemplate the idea of MNF as a possibility.

There is a document on the Internet I first read in 2000 entitled 'nuclear fusion in molecular systems' by three chemistry professors. It is only in last 8 years that papers on Molecular Nuclear Fusion on Blogger have overtaken this original seminal paper.

High Intensity UltraSound (150 W 40 kHz) apply it to a cancerous organ will cure their cancer at one appointment. With no drug use. All other diseases of age will respond to HIUS.

Every biological organism on earth does Molecular Nuclear Fusion! Getting energy from the nuclear fusion of hydrogen atoms bound up in water. It should therefore be no surprise that ultrasound induces nuclear fusion.
$H_2O \rightarrow He + O + E^2 + L + X\text{-ray}$

I know that I have already mentioned this equation elsewhere in this book. But I am so proud of the thinking behind it! The amount of Molecular Nuclear Fusion ultrasound induces is linked to the system pressure.

This is why diesel engines outperform petrol engines. This is also why High Intensity UltraSound causes the cell contents of the pressurised cancer cell, like cancers to expand and boil. While not affecting normal body cells around and in front of it.

Petrol will spontaneously combust, but a higher pressure than diesel, if we inject the fuel via a turbulent injection system injection pressure them a diesel system is produced. Fluid turbulence is the catalyst to engineering Molecular Nuclear Fusion.

This why bacteria that produce methane and helium gases! At higher pressures this methane ends up as methyl hydrate. This white solid is on ocean floors around the world. We can robot mine it.

And when we reduce the applied pressure get methane and water. Methyl hydrate is the metastable CH_5OH. At one atmosphere pressure we get CH_4 and H_2O.

The methane is basically natural gas with no sulphur in! In Brazil there reduce the tax on low sulphur fuels, but ended up having to augment the sulphur in the air otherwise crop yields were reduced.

That is why global warming is such rubbish! By the day global photosynthesis on land and in the seas converts additional CO_2 and SO_2 into additional plant growth. Global Warming was rubbish by nuclear power to try and justify more toxic nuclear fission plants.

In the Jurassic age there were no fossil fuels. 85% more life on land, sea levels 60 metres lower but the level of carbon dioxide in the air was still reduced to a 4 parts per million trace by photosynthesis. Twice today;s global average.

Levels in an ice age, in the polar air, are back at 4ppm. Air temperature at -50^pC.

Burning fossil fuels so does not increase the level of carbon dioxide in the air. It increases the amount of life on earth!

Animals only evolved to metabolise oxygen and carbohydrates, at the end of the Permian was a carbon crisis. Too little CO_2 - 90% of life on Earth died, Biggest mass extinction in history.

Where the evolution of photosynthesis reduces free carbon dioxide are to half today's present two parts per million. 90% of life on earth died. Ever since animals and plants have been in a dynamic balance.

More carbon dioxide results in the restoration of life to the surface of the earth. It does not affect the gas composition of the air. So there is no weather effect! Maybe after this book, I will write one about nuclear climate fiction. This is rather more important! Already written and corrected. My publisher LOVES it.

Back to the production of ultrasound : of particular interest is the concentration effect produced by the guide tube the emitter sits at the base of. We don't want focused ultrasound! We could use a guide tube to produce a concentrated cone of ultrasound fire centimetres beyond the emitter.

This would produce too focused an effect for us! We would prefer the slowly diverging cone of ultrasound in HIUS. Ultrasound will be dumped from 150 W to 90 W as it passes through tissues around and in the body. For lung cancer the chest is a major concern to the use of HIUS.

2013, I used High Intensity UltraSound to cure lung cancer at 1 session. So I was wrong to be concerned. And 80% of cancers out there are lung cancer. Now totally curable - 1 session of High Intensity UltraSound at home.

Ultrasound does travel through body tissues. Not as effectively as bass sound! 25 Hz will travel quite happily through feet of sound insulation. This is why discos tend to be sited away from populated areas.

They were trying to cite one in Trafford Park only 2 miles away from where I move; at media village by the BBC in England! The BBC could afford the expensive lawyers to fight the traffic application. It did not get planning consent.

The initial planning outline does not cost money to fight! As I know from my work on the housing development in Bury. The way that builders work, is to look at the initial objections, modify their proposals and keep coming back until the planning application is approved.

The proposed Disco in Trafford Park hopefully have just given in! There must be other industrial areas that are not next to the £140 million development that is a Media City. The builders will be well advised to look elsewhere!

I have mentioned elsewhere that we could 120 W 40 kHz. Now state of the art is 8W 1MHz. Will cure all cancers out there. It will not result in the person coughing up blood for three days, or ever again! As is the way with active lung cancer.

Above 90 W the pressurise cancer cells fragment. We use 40 kHz as ultrasonic carpet cleaners have found this frequency causes the boil off, of water sprayed on the ground. This instantaneous boiling is what we want to induce in cancer cells.

I knew about ultrasound boiling water in 1986! But I was away being married and working in IT. I trusted other scientists to follow this up. Certainly in 2000 it was germane for me to investigate around the department of Engineering Materials at Sheffield University.

No policy advise was given to this, as all chemical laboratories in universities around the world were so dependent on the money they acquired from the funding agencies to study global warming. Annoyingly the world has started cooling naturally in 1995.

Hence the sudden ending of my P_hD. 2004 was a bad hurricane year-exactly on the natural schedule. Not man-made Climate Change, natural weather.

Hence the sudden change in nuclear PR to man made climate change. Trouble is, this totally ignores global photosynthesis. And Global Warming was 'true science without doubt'. Now in a cooling world - just so wrong.

The trace of carbon dioxide we see in the air since after the Permian age, is directly controlled by global photosynthesis. In the Jurassic this was four parts per million. Since the little ice age carbon dioxide has been limited to 2ppm.

The the climate pundits are especially annoyed when you remind them that there were three natural ice ages in the Jurassic age: CO_2 doubled - at 4 parts per million. Sea levels 60 metres lower. 85% more life on earth. And less fossil fuels!

Photosynthesis was less efficient back then. So the same level of carbon dioxide in the air as he saw here in the little ice age. Just as man started burning the fossil fuels. The level of carbon dioxide in the air halved as the ice and snow receded.

Much to the annoyance of ill educated climate pundits, carbon dioxide levels only rise in natural ice ages. In the three natural ice ages of the Jurassic, carbon dioxide levels rose.

Just as life on earth had increased. In exactly the opposite fashion to the predictions of man made global warming and climate change.

In a warm period there was 85% more life on land. Sea levels 60 metres lower. In the Jurassic ice ages free carbon dioxide levels rose to eight parts per million.

By now you should be wondering where the ideas of global warming came from? Obviously the individuals involved have no basic grasp of photosynthesis, no historical data, are not large research contracts for nuclear power.

Interesting, as nuclear power;s plant turn over, makes them the 4th biggest source of CO2. Natural lightening and plant life main sources of No/NO2. Diesel engines not important at all. Petrol engines not important either - though a bigger source of all emissions.

In the major ice age of the Cretaceous into the Permian, which lasted 1000 years, there was five times as much carbon dioxide in the air as today. We can safely conclude carbon dioxide is a climate follower. And has no forcing effect on the weather.

The data on the lower infrared permeability of CO_2 only cuts in at 2%! 10,000 times more than nature allows in the global air. A climate pundit quite happily told me there was 20% carbon dioxide in the global air.

Carbon dioxide is toxic to all animal life at 8%! Oxygen is at 20%. CO_2 is at a static 0.0002%-and has been static for the last 200 years.

The mineral and ice core records over last 100 million years recalls the carbon dioxide rises 4 years after a natural ice age has commenced. It does not cause the ice age! And certainly does not cause global warming.

The academics who generated ¼ century of fantastic incomes from talking absolute biological rubbish should NEVER have been in eduction. There is pretence they they understand the majority of biology. They had no basic grasp of the carbon cycle. These people should not be in the media or education.

The global climate is exclusively controlled by solar cycles! Carbon dioxide drives biology. Nuclear power drives global death. Nuclear fission is simpler at causing death on a continental scale. The least green technology conceivable. I really must write this up in a book!

It is at a sublime coincidence, that ultrasound induces fatal levels of biological molecular nuclear fusion specifically in cancer infected cells. Only bystander damage goes on in body cells. Your own body does nuclear fusion. Cancer exposed to HIUS does such fatal levels of it - limited to cancer etc. cells..

Ultrasound causes no long term side effects. Only doing stander, and easily fixed damage to body cells. And in time the blood loss will be made good by the intact stem cells.

And the cancer will be gone. Both the primarily, and any secondaries. With no drug use or surgery. No failing, expensive painful treatment. A total cure. No Doctor or hospital/drug company required.

And without the major income stream of drug companies. HIUS will also clear heart disease, diabetes, MS, and arthritis, IBS and all infections including the common cold. Almost unnoticed the world has changed.

And that drug companies are trying to suppress the news that all the diseases of age are now routinely curable. They never in their wildest dreams thought this would happen! Biochemistry is totally sidelined. Criminal medicine for 16 years. All prescribing Doctors, and their drug firms struck off - out of medicine.

No failing treatments that are expensive, painful and ultimately fatal system - as today! A one appointment total cure. The drug companies are adaptive.

I anticipate they will start offering HIUS regimes to clear away cessated cells. And change human ageing. After all, they are licensed for medical treatments. Home cure is best and cheapest. No health insurance required.

We do not paying the drug companies massive amounts of money, to give us failing painful treatments for diseases they do not understand. We do not want extra years of ill heath and disability.

We pay them to cure us. That is the last thing they wish to do! They would prefer our to treat us. Where we die, our place is taken by other poor individuals.

I heard today that MS drugs have gone up in price by a factor 20. But no great reason. Only to replace the lost income drug companies experience now that cancer and MS are routinely curable. 120 W 40 kHz/8W 1MHz

HIUS apply it to each side of the head for ½ a minute will cure the viral/bacterial rump that causes MS.

After a serious illness a fragment of a virus can be copied out as a pathogen leader. This colonise the myelin sheath around neurons: bacteria gravitate towards the CNS-where the immune system has restricted access.

When the main bacteria is cleared, the bacterial/viral rump is left behind. Making inappropriate interleukin two! Pathogen leaders from the MS mess with the efficiency of the immune system. Over stimulated and untargeted macrophages crashing around doing damage, and make life easier for a pathogen.

Professor Howard Weiner of Harvard University medical school told me about the inappropriate production of IL-2 being important to MS! During a relapse of MS, we can give additional immune action.

Now be inappropriate production of IL-2 just improves the efficiency of the immune system clearing the bacterial rump. But if we had IL-4, we would cause the B cells to make and action the active human antibody to all viral and bacterial rumps in the body.

If we apply reduced power HIUS the to the head, we cause the overinflated bacterial rumps to fragment! The oligonucleotides repair the myelin sheath. All the Astra sites replace the damaged neurons.

Now we have fully cleared the MS in five weeks. With no biochemical pills used. Cured. Not treated! So no biochemistry is ever required in MS. Professor Weiner will already have found new areas to study-he is a clever guy. Wrong again - he retired as he heard about my ideas.

My old girlfriend developed MS after a bad mumps infection! In my youth I have such an infection-but do not get MS!

A quick course of ultrasound sessions would have seen her right! Isn't High Intensity UltraSound a wonderful thing! Certainly, if you have MS today, you need a medical friend to apply ultrasound to you. Drugs do nothing.

Come on medics, get the HIUS kits and get curing. Start saving lives. MS like heart disease is not a big problem. Stop trying to earn an income stream from it! Just cure the disease.

Drug companies are meant to be in the business of extending human health. They actually extend the years of painful, expensive and ultimately fatal years of disability.

The drug companies are the merchants of death. Like some anti hero of a spy novel. Only better paid! 'Doctor Death is thinking of new, horrible ways to kill you!'

The FDA and NICE do not have to licence ultrasound! In large measure because mankind has been utilising it since the 1950s. Then for shipbuilding and metallurgical uses.

But it is more effective at clearing the diseases of age. Just no biologists have never considered it. This was out of their field of expertise. It just happened to be in two of my area of training and work.

Drug companies were quite happy to use lower power ultrasound to image cancer and there tumours. Increasing the applied power of the ultrasound results in the structures causing the diseases of age to explosively fragment. And this cures the disease itself. With no surgery or drug use.

HIUS has no affect on regular body tissues. People can experiment with it, and do no harm! Utilising ultrasound the individual finds that magically the diseases of age are cleared.

This is why it does not require FDA approval. Try it! Cheapest source, an 8W 1MHz ultrasound massage device. A medically licensed beauty device - save for home use.

The worst that can happen is that you do not get better. In actual fact you will recover completely from the diseases of age.

This was the big income area for the drug company is. I await seeing what they will do! Cancer, heart disease, diabetes, mental health problems all cured. This is all they said they ever wanted!

The occupational health date for last 60 years have shown that the diseases of age affect Manual workers as they cease to be exposed to ultrasound. Promotion or retirement are such a massive changes in the environment; but all scientists overlooked this affect!

Putting the medical affects down to less exercise, increased smoking and eating. And the body itself be less vital - so important? The data out there- though we could only see the affect once we knew exactly what we're looking for. When we knew the answer, it was obvious!

Coughing up blood will sop as you cure lung cancer. Patients with lung cancer are used a coughing up blood. Other patients may be quite alarmed. 1 application of High Intensity UltraSound - no more coughing up blood, or persist ant pain.

After 1 application of High Intensity UltraSound all such discharges will cease! Presumably will also see tenderness and inflammation of the cancerous organ, will instantly subside. 1 minute of High Intensity UltraSound is the total cure! The growing cancer itself under biochemical pills, is vastly more uncomfortable and painful.

Gastrointestinal cancers will result in darkened stools for three days. It is unlikely that anybody would notice unless they inspected the toilet carefully after use. This is the modus operendus of the Germans. High Intensity UltraSound for 1 minute to the affected gut - no more cancers.

So HIFU cures cancer. By inducing nuclear fusion in cancer cells. Dr. MatZinger said my big contribution to the future was molecular nuclear fusion. Presumably she is slightly extrapolating my educational background. One smart lady!

When she told me, I thought this meant I would cure global warming. But nature did that in 1995! The climate is now in a cooling phase. I never dreamt that Molecular Nuclear Fusion applied to cancer, would produce a one appointment cure. Everything is connected! Everything is a system. The weather and immunology are two obvious systems.

If she had not told me this personally, I have probably never would have worked in this area! There again, my P_hD colleague at Sheffield University may have influenced by an academic interests. Or felt I could fill in gaps in the total picture.

But around the world there are 400,000 scientists with the required ultrasound experience. Academic institutions with a higher level experience in engineering- know all the basics of HIFU. It is very rare though for your mentor to encourage you to free think! Thank you professor Argent.

Cancer cells are normal body cells, with pathogen additions at the end of the DNA. In a structure called the endogenous retro virus. Medics do like their Greek and Latin mixed root names. Or just plain gobbledegook.

To gain a vitality advantage all pathogens cells are over inflated compared to flaccid body cells. They demand and get extra blood supplies using endothelial growth factor. This grows additional blood vessels into the viral or cancer body.

Bacterial cells are just free swimming and overinflated structures. Within their minimal cell wall provided by the ever over helpful B cells.

I knew that ultrasound causes water at atmospheric pressure to boil almost instantly. I also knew that the pressurised diesel cycle apple formed the lower power petrol cycle-even though diesel fuel it was a lower energy fuel.

Time for a chemical equation! Sorry there are no checks in this novel, I do not find anything about cancer remotely funny.

$C_m(H_2O)_n + pO_2 \to nHe + mCO_2 + qO_3 + E + \gamma$

$C_m(H_2O)_n$ is a chemical equation for hydrocarbon. And yes I realise that q is related to p and m. But it really is not important to the story. We get out helium gas. Of which there is no chemical source! From both diesel and petrol engines.

The CO_2 produced is metabolised by global photosynthesis to increase life on earth. Emissions have no effect on the weather. The trace of carbon dioxide left in the air by photosynthesis has been static since levels fell at the end of the little ice age. Then they were higher! 4ppm. In an ice age.

Man made global warming and climate change are oxymoron devised by the diseased minds of the paid stooges to nuclear power. Another one of my little areas, that I will have discussed further in this book.

The Point I was trying to make here, is not actually contained in the equations! The production of helium is linked to the pressure of combustion. If the engine is now run at higher pressure, so they do more molecular nuclear fusion. They produce more motive energy.

So we never get to cancer cells. Dividing uncontrollably like amoeba. This is single cell type division, to avoid scrutiny by the immune system.

The dendrite mesh stops any inappropriate cell division so viruses and cancer divides in a single cell way. This has ramifications! The body only permits such behaviour as it is intrinsic to live childbirth. A growing mass of tissue that is half not the mother.

The placenta damp down the mother's immune system-so pregnancy is the peak period for the mother to have bad viruses and cancer. We are reptilian viral symbiosis. We only exist because a distant ancestor had a bad virus. Further back, we laid eggs.

And the trick for single cell division colonised some cells in the mother's womb as the pathogen leader. Bacteria and viruses take away, but they also give. Your colon reclaims the water from your food using bacteria. They are better at this than the human body cells.

We are all here because of the distant earth past. The tree rats, our distant ancestors, came from the reptilian line, and went on to the creator all mammals including the giant apes. Because of some viral genome.

Reptiles still exist, in energy scarce environments! Another trick we acquired from pathogens is that warm blooded nature! The mitochondria that perform this trick hold their DNA away from the genetic DNA. They were a captured life form - from our food.

Some scientists argue this is because of captive free swimming bacteria. I don't think so! Mitochondrial activity is to do biological molecular nuclear fusion: $CO_2 + 3H_2O \rightarrow He + CH_4 + O. + E + \gamma$

Some of you will notice this is the energy creation scheme that causes cancer cells to boil off. Mitochondria do it as a much lower level! Every cell in your body is supported by biological molecular nuclear fusion.

Cancer cells are greedy! Their mitochondria do more life Molecular Nuclear Fusion anyway. This is why cancer cells are overinflated, under supported and warm.

Neither viruses nor bacteria have to survive in the world full of ultrasound! Manual workers suffer fewer cancers and the diseases of age because of the daily air exposure to ultrasound. I only realise that as I investigated HIUS and cancer. It is easy one to know, if you know the answer.

Suddenly cancer cells do fatal amounts of Molecular Nuclear Fusion. Very vital - stealing all the body's food.

The important element of this story is the disguised nature of necrosis that goes on in cancer tumours. Soft body cancers respond to the same ideas. I'll get back to them if I remember! So the cell damage going on in a cancer tumour is not seen by the clustering dendrites.

Luckily I had training in metallurgical ultrasound. And following my head injury, my then girlfriend had mortal sclerosis, and so I developed an interest in medicine. Dr. MatZinger transformed this in two an interest in cancer and the diseases of age. Which includes MS, heart disease, diabetes. Cancer and IBS.

Really this is at the limit on my understanding. I needed some medical input. A useful description of HIUS is 150 W 40 kHz, or now 8W 1MHz. High Intensity Focused Ultrasound is High Intensity UltraSound applied through a thin tube 10cm centimetres long.

This can be deduced by any engineer with an interest in ultrasound and access to the Internet to do their own research! Google 'toxicity ultrasound' and then 'ultrasonic carpet cleaners'. The latter work by boiling off water sprayed onto the carpet. Which is what we want to induce in cancer cells.

This is one description of HIUS. 90 W/cm^2 40kHz should be toxic to the pressurise cancer cells. They lack support from the dendrite mesh. But body tissues attenuate ultrasound. So 150 W ultrasound enters a body, not leaves at 120 W!

The Florida connection

The medics in Florida and California have a large interest in age and cancer. Dr. MatZinger was interested in me working in California with Dr. Mel Cohn. If he ever bothered to get in touch, I now have a useful stuff to talk with him about.

In 2001 I sent my thoughts on ultrasound to my medical contacts. At the NI H, Cambridge University and Harvard University. There was talk about me doing a Ph.D. At the latter two. But my master's degree in engineering is not sufficient to do a medical Ph.D..

Which leaves me free to sing for iTunes with my folk group: they are called OldSorts. They used to be

Odsoccs, and the videos are still on YouTube. Fun, but it doesn't save life on earth! X-factor - who knows.

2002 the Moffitt cancer centre in Florida tried out High Intensity UltraSound on prostate cancer tumours. They found it was a one appointment cure. With no drug use or surgery is appropriate!

The ultrasound they did not just image the cancer tumours! The ultrasound causes the tumour to release nuclear radiation.

$H_2O+US \rightarrow He+O+E^2+X\text{-ray}$

The emission of gamma wave/X-ray radiation and production of helium gas is symptomatic of a nuclear action. And there is no source of nuclear fission specific to cancer cells.

We are causing the pressurised cancer cell contents to do biological molecular nuclear fusion. Physicists would be intrigued by the production of nuclear radiation. Medics were just happy that photographic film got an image with no light.

We don't apply X rays or gamma waves! The ultrasound stimulates the production of nuclear radiation from cancer cells. That is remarkable! But more important is the production of heat -the E^2.

Low power ultrasound warms up cancer cells by 4° C. Body cells by 0.1° C. Totally insignificant environmental noise!

HIUS causes only cancer cells to heat up to 60°C - and die. At 120° C they explosively fragment. You would think that cell death was sufficient! The immune system clears away death cells, so most of the cancer cells will be removed.

Simplistic! The explosive fragmentation damages body cells to within a two cell radius of the cancer tumour. These body cells are on the dendrite mesh. The dendrites are aware of the cell damage.

They are also see this novel DNA/RNA in the blood stream. They make and action the specific antibodies to the dangerous cell type. Including the six common enzymes to all viruses and cancer-and the five common with bacterial infections.

The body now sees cancer as dangerous. And it is removed throughout the body! All remaining cells in the primary and all secondary classes anywhere in the body.

From one application of HIFU. With no cancer traces left behind, and no cancer surgery: Which is medical medieval mutilation!

Cancer drugs are over specific, too expensive, only treat the cancer, and ultimately allow the cancer to kill you. Through the inappropriate growth of an differentiated tissues starving other cells to death!

HIV and other weak infections

HIV is not a good virus. It falls below immune scrutiny as it causes no cell damage. Just like cancer! Even minor cell damage causes the immune system to launch an immune assault against a pathogen (with a head start).

Once cell damage has been detected, the antigen presenting centres (APCs) of the body make and actions the specific human antibodies. It turns IL-1 into two lots of the effective IL-1+. The immune system can even eat bone, so must be turned off to allow live childbirth.

This is why sharks get cancer. But egg-laying reptiles do not! Live childbirth and cancer are linked. IL-1+ makes IL-2…21. My master's degree was in systems work. Infections do not initiate the immune system for three days.

There is no reason to wait for an immune action. We have a biochemical industry that is perfectly capable of mass producing human antibody pills.

Will return to my point about there being five common enzymes to all infections! Anyone antibody to these enzymes will cure all infections. Pathogens avoid antibody production by avoiding significant cell damage for three days.

We can just avoid the need for cell damage! We give a combined drip of IL-2 and IL-4. The IL-4 makes the human antibody to non-native genome anywhere in the body! Even cancer is sampled by the B cells.

They look at the antigen presenting surface for novel enzymes. Around the site of cell damage. HIV and SARs-as well as cancer do not do cell damage.

So there is no natural production of IL-4. Or your own the immune system would eat any embryo in the world.

If the individual is not pregnant, and we gave IL-4 by direct the liver, B cells, dendrites and APC cells make the active antibody. And drop it into the bloodstream. Which in time it will be cleared by the liver. This was my idea about cancer 8 years ago. That did work!

However, if we have IL-2 about the T cells cluster around the APCs, and get loaded with the antibody! They transporting it to the macrophages, who then go off and engulf the target cell. The antibody in actioned!

I have been wittering on about this idea for nine years. The drug companies are making too much money selling failing treatments.   So how absolutely no interest in an effective cure to HIV, cancer and the other diseases of age!

We have removed the need for cell damage! So, of course, we cure cancer. But we also cure HIV and the rest. Which displaying the novel antigens in the antigen presenting surface, even if they do not cause cell damage!

The body seas the IL-s in the blood, and assumes cell damage is occurring elsewhere in the body! If it was the local APCs would damp down the immune system by excreting IL-10. This system does not always work, as people still develop allergies.

Where a harmless substance is linked to cell damage being done by another agent! Mostly to heat and substances, or rings on the fingers.

A way he to remove these allergies is to invest the electric substance in harmless fat. We then have of course of injections. Where we inject increasing amounts of the fat containing the allergic response disappears.

As they bypass the stomach, we do not have cell damage! Heating and digesting food breaks up the animal matter, and this acts as a marker for cell damage which is seen by the immune system. The body works hard to stop this immune action! Which causes a lot of gastrointestinal cancers.

Injecting the allergic substance gradually deletes the T memory cells-immune system T cells carry the memory of the danger of this substance. Without medical speak; we just remove the allergy!

By a drip of interleukin two and four we induce the allergy response to weak viruses like HIV etc.. It turns out that strawberry allergies teach us of useful stuff. The allergic response has the potential to cure all cancers humans get.

Because the HIV he does not actually do damage, the allergic response is removed every time they capture the disease. So we need to cure the HIV again! This is the way with cancers! There is nothing to stop you from getting cancer again. We have to cure heat infection and must prevent the diseases of age occurring.

This was written before I found out about High-Intensity UltraSound. Which turns out to be the best home cure to all cancers, When a person is given the drip of IL-2&4, their own immune systems produce the human antibody to HIV. Pills of this substance will cure other instances of the disease.

Obviously, ½ a minute of High-Intensity UltraSound to each side of the chest, fragments the HIV virus, and stimulates the production of the human antibody to cure all HIV – no biochemistry involved.

If you do not desist from dangerous behaviour, releasing use all the HIV pills or High-Intensity UltraSound is appropriate! The same approach will work for all types of cancer. All cancers cured on demand.

My top viewed video on YouTube had 26,000 hits as I am writing this! By the time you read, it should be over 100,000. No drug company is interested in curing anything. Let alone HIV or cancer. They are interested in making money.

They will only be interested in treating people to stop them from developing the diseases of age if there is money in it! Will no longer be any more money made from failing treatments of the developed cancer.

Cancer cure

This is why he bought this book! A software version on my words will cost under two UK pounds. A paper back around £10 UK pounds I thought the paperback version is going to cost you the price of 3 packets of cigarettes. For the narrative that will save your life! What a bargain.

Not buying their 3 packets of cigarettes might stop you developing lung cancer. Annoyingly the ideas in this book will cure lung cancer. I still think it is a deity stupid disease inducing addiction.

The pressurised cancer cells are dividing uncontrollably. But not doing any cell damage seen by the clustering dendrites. All the cell necrosis caused by the rapid budding of body cells is engulfed by surrounding cancer cells. So drug tolerance to the drugs marketed by drug companies spreads through the cancer rapidly!

Then we apply ultrasound. Low power makes the cancer tumour light up the nuclear radiation, and heat up by a few degrees.

We apply HIUS to the cancer tumour. Suddenly that E^2-the energy gets to be very important! Rather than just a few degrees, the cancer heats up past 60° C. Body cells by 0.8° C. So a body cells are totally unaffected by HIUS. Cancer cells boil.

Radiology departments the world over should have HIUS machines. As should every GP surgery. When ultrasound has located a cancer tumour, they are applying a quick buzz of HIFU for 1 minute.

Cancer, diabetes, heart disease and infective disease itself - which gets to be the minor key to all conditions.

No pill swallowing required! We are totally insensitive to ultrasound. 40 kHz is way above the hearing range of people. We can't hear even over 20 kHz when we are young. Bats came hear up to 150 kHz. Not 1MHz.

To treat cancer in bats, we not need need to equip them with little hearing projections. Hearing does decrease in age, so in your sixty's you struggle to hear above 12 kHz.

A more perfect hearing top frequency may be 350 kilohertz. So there is no obstacle to zoos employing ultrasound kit at 160 kHz. Our main interest is in curing human cancers and diseases of age though!

The primary cancer tumour is decimated! And the immune system launches an effective immune assault on that cancer secondaries. Including production of IL-2&4. Ultrasound causes the body to produce IL-1+ and IL-2...21.

So the positive feedback system used by the immune system man is for the the immune assault throughout the body to clear the cancer. An immune action in one area of the body becomes body wide.

The body can learn novel genome, but not if we give the IL-2&4 from a biochemical drip. Evolution never considered that a realistic possibility. For centuries drug companies could have produced the human antibodies to cancer.

By stimulating the immune system with the cytokines IL-2&4. Maybe I am being a bit harsh. Certainly these chemicals have been known about since the 1950s. The human antibodies are natural chemicals - not patentable. So there was never any money to be made from producing them.

These drugs would have cured all infections, cancer and the diseases of age. Again the drug companies are not in business to be optimistic. They can only exist while they make money. Ultrasound is going to seriously disrupt their income stream. They will adapt, to selling ultrasound regimes to keep a person fit and healthy. But all the Doctors are struck off - along with the nurses,

People will not be immortal. There are other diseases out there waiting to cull us. The words on my grandmother, who died from dementia 4 years ago.

In my chapter about HIV, I lamented the lack of cell damage means every instance of the infection will require a new course of human antibody fuels to clear it. The drug companies are not in mourning. They depend on it! But now we use a buzz of HIUS to stimulate production of antibodies - not on popping expensive pills.

So with cancer! Every time a person contracts an infection they will require a course of human antibody pills to cure the infection - a buzz of High Intensity UltraSound! Or they will require a course of pills to clear the cancer that it helps create! All of the world requires application of HIUS. Just the best medicine.

The kits to utilising ultrasound to remove wrinkles (and the diseases of age) are available on E bay for 13 UK pounds. At the correct power and frequency.

Certainly kits which do should be available all over the world for a modest price.

GP surgeries think they require more expensive medically licensed kits. These are on sale for $10,000. The manufacturers cannot be serious! The kits should retail for $25. And manufactured to withstand constant use.

As he infective disease leaves behind, as pathogen leaders, the seed corns for cancer. Cure the infection rapidly, no cancers form.

The antibody pills and High Intensity UltraSound kits will cure infections and stop cancer. And be required often. To a world population of 10 billion! Though we cannot use the pills with a woman who may be pregnant.

And no doubt there are religious people who would rather die than use biochemistry or technology. This after all is what biochemistry has worked so hard towards for so many years! An agonising death of the innocents.

Soft body cancers &MS

Is very related to HIV. They display novel antigens, but like all cancers do not do any cell damage. A drip of the IL-2&4 will produce the active human antibody to clear such structures from the body.

A ½ minute buzz of High Intensity UltraSound to each side of the scull will produce the active human antibody to MS.

As with the other diseases of age, the pathogen leaders of infective disease accumulate genome in cessated cells that causes cancer. With MS we get inappropriate production of interleukin two. In soft body cancer they are budding of body cells results in the liberation of rapidly dividing blood cells.

Usually blood cells are produced by cell budding in the bone marrow. I think it likely that there cancer mother cell is a cessated cells within the liver or bone marrow.

A buzz of High Intensity UltraSound will clear it. Ultrasound scans will show the location.

With MS a bacterial rump colonising in the fatty sheath around neurons. The immune system ignores such structures until the patient is ill. Even then the immune system is too targeted on the infection sites, and makes them ineffective attempt to clear the bacterial rump.

With leukaemia we can also employ HIUS. Applying the ultrasound to a major body long bone for 1 minute. The soft body cancer will fragment. Distributing novel genome where the B cells can see it! The B cells make an action the specific human antibody to the soft body cancer.

MS hides in the CNS. Where the immune system has restricted access! There is no local antigen presenting centre in the brain. If we cause the bacterial rump to fragment, the B cells are allowed into the brain area, and make and action the specific human antibody to clear MS.

At least in MS the static bacterial/viral rumps are target for our ultrasound. But the brain area is usually hidden off from the immune system! Which is why brain cancer, along with MS are tricky problems.

But the skull is no barrier to ultrasound. We require no brain surgery, we just have to live with the extra attenuation caused by the skull bones. To ultrasound the skull hardly exists at all! It involved as a physical barrier. So on sound passes straight through it.

With leukaemia the B cells act as antigen presenting centres. We lack a target organ to ultrasound. But the flowing blood gives us a target for the HIUS. The body requires only to see the lose DNA. Then it gets its act together! And clears the dangerous structure from the body.

I would like to take the opportunity to mention multiple sclerosis. Hear my thanks go to Professor Weiner at Harvard Medical school, who helped me formulate my ideas about pathogen leaders - first suggested by professor Fossil.

Mr MatZinger wanted me to do a PHD at Harvard. But medicine is a closed shop! And my master's degree in engineering and metallurgy do not facilitate such a move.

MS is caused by pathogen leaders left behind from serious infections making inappropriate interleukin two. IL-2 on its own over stimulates the white blood cells. But does not clear the bacterial rump.

The bacterial rump here colonises the myelin sheath. And the immune system destroys the functioning of the neuron as it makes them ineffective attempt to clear the infestations.

So close but no cancer causing cigar. A drip of interleukin four during an MS relapse will clear the infection. As to repairing the damage, see my chapter on repairing the cells of age.

Heart Disease

Here the pathogen rump is another bacterial infestation. This time colonising the fatty sheaths along the coronary arteries. This was is why the naïve think Statins might have a role. They do not. Adding just 4 days to a heart patient's life.

Medics have found that the bacterial rump is also around the kidneys - as these have the major role in controlling the blood sugar level and pressure.

Both directly via a nerve and admire production of the enzyme rennin. The bacterial rump around the kidneys causes secondary heart disease.

The use of High Intensity UltraSound on the kidneys has led to a 100% cure rate of secondary coronary heart disease. I will return to this point at the end of this article: let us proceed with the rump on the coronary arteries.

High Intensity UltraSound to the top left of the chest clears primary heart diseases. No medication needed, or helpful.

A drip of IL-2&4 will sort out all rump problems in the body. But drug companies have shown less than zero interest in this idea.

As I say elsewhere throughout his tone, drug companies are not interested in cures. They can only make money from treatments. HIUS is an act just one time cure of the diseases of age.

Are the drug companies nimble footed enough to produce a viable business, before the engineers get their ultrasound and act together. There is certainly going to be a lot of healthy competition in the HIUS market.

All I can say is bring it on! Applying High Intensity UltraSound to the coronary arteries causes the troublesome bacterial rumps to fragment. They may induce an immune action. Resultingly we clear all the specific pathogen rumps of that type from the body.

Heart disease is no more! This was the big income stream of cancers was removed gradually. In 2002 the Moffitt cancer centre started curing prostate cancer at one application of HIUS. Cancer was then cured by the physical method. Biochemistry looked so dated.

It was over expensive, two specific and in competition with the compatible drugs produced in India and China. These drugs were developed by the drug companies 25 years previously.

I have seen media articles documenting the lack of progress made in biochemistry by the U.S. drug companies over the last decade. Presumably because they realized with the ultrasound work, cancer was cured!

They could have saved serious lives, if they have worked mainly to accomplish this. They fought a massive rearguard action, to protect their dwindling income. Hence the chapter Xi bankruptcy filed by drug companies!

Astra Zeneca was the world's wealthiest company. Last I heard, it was no longer even in the top 10. But the time the world learned about High Intensity UltraSound -

from reading this book and others they will no longer be in the top 100.

Heart disease is cured by HIUS -The fragments of the bacterial rumps are removed by the liver. All rump structures are tiny, and the body is set up to remove strands of loose DNA. The same argument applies with MS! Once the immune system is targeted, the bacterial rump is history.

The damage to the brain by MS, strokes and head/spinal injuries should be repaired by the Astrocites- the brain stem cells, activated by HIUS. This is the area that Professor Weiner should have been working on.

Overinflated structures or bacterial Colonies with minimal cell walls accumulate in the human body with age and infections. Luckily all such pathogen rumps are over inflated and will fragment explosively on application of HIFU.

Medics have tried out HIUS on coronary heart disease. I would expect HIUS apply it to the coronary arteries to correct for primary coronary heart disease. Clearing the bacterial rump which colonise the fatty plaques around the coronary arteries.

Total cure to heart disease using High Intensity UltraSound, medically published in a 20 patient double blind trial 2012.

They have already experienced a 100% cure rate of secondary coronary heart disease applying the ultrasound to the kidneys. A person with coronary heart disease should ultrasound the coronary arteries and the kidneys.

Since our originally wrote this piece, I have learned some basic medicine: It is not the job of our heart to regulate blood pressure. That task is delegated to the kidneys. Which have a major nerve running to the heart! They also produce the enzyme rennin to increase the blood pressure.

For secondary coronary heart disease - HIUS will clear the bacterial rumps around the kidneys that interferes with the regulatory system!

I would expect the rumps to be making inappropriate endocrine signals that are picked up and acted on by the heart. Or directly interfere with the functioning of the kidneys. Or the production of Rennin of course.

As mentioned above ; medics applied HIUS to the kidneys and cleared the secondary coronary heart disease. At one application. With no biochemical involvement;-no pills or surgery is appropriate.

So applying HIUS to the kidneys clears the inappropriately high blood pressure this disease is characterised by.

As I have been saying for last decade, a drip of IL-2&4 will produce the human antibody to clear heart disease. With one course of pills!

Diabetes

Yet again is caused by another viral rump infestations. I tend to think like cancer it is a viral rump.

Some basic medical work established this. But no university or medical company are ever going to publish certainty. There is no income stream to be derived.

As some were lodged in my mind in a published autopsy of a diabetes patient. There were hardened structures in the pancreas. Just as heart disease has hardened structures along the coronary arteries. A quick buzz of HIFU will clear up the viral rumps. External to the bottom right of the chest for 1 minute.

Yes he really is that simple! The money to be made is from preventing cancer and the diseases of age. Curing them once they have happened is not that hard! But they are inconvenient and painful conditions to extremes.

This will cure Type 1&2 diabetes. Again my proof reader has a vested interest in diabetes! As it formed his nursing dissertation before he graduated. Time, events and life moves on. I have lost two grandfathers and one grandmother to diabetes!

Type 1, 1 minute of High Intensity UltraSound. Type 2, ½ minute. 8W 1MHz ultrasound.

If only I had known then, what I know now! Is only I had avoided driving home the night of my car accident. Hindsight is 2020 annoyingly!

Things have moved on. Biochemistry has dictated for too long that medicine is theirs. The NI H has used biochemical work on curing type 1 diabetes. HIUS provides an almost trivial cure to this condition.

The biochemical cure to type 2 has been out for around 2 years. Both cures use expensive Bio chemical pills. A buzz of ultrasound in the GP surgery will cost 10p.

Since I write this, they have tried out HIUS on diabetes! But they did not apply it to the pancreas. The organ that regulates blood sugar levels is the kidney. So they applied HIUS to kidneys. I did the pancreas, and cured it.

I think for patients with little type 1 diabetes-my ideas about HIFU and the pancreas apply also to type 2 diabetes and the kidneys. The medics tried it with the kidneys and found they got a 100% cure rate!

It turns out there is a bacterial rump in the fatty deposits around the kidneys. HIUS removes this! And suddenly their blood auger regulation returns to normal.

Diabetes patients also tend to suffer from coronary heart disease. And guess what! HIUS apply it to the kidneys clears secondary coronary heart disease.

One of my friends had type two diabetes. I have lost non blood relatives to all versions of diabetes previously.

I thought the disease was caused by left over pathogen leader forming a viral rump in the pancreas.

My nursing friend confirmed the hardened white structures were visible and low power ultrasound scan. Eureka.

So I applied high intensity ultrasound to my friend with diabetes. I was using a personal ultrasound massage device at 150 W 40 kHz. Now 8W 1MHz - 30 times cheaper to use and more effective.

Technically the Americans term this HIUS. The variety of ultrasound the Moffitt employed before HIFU.

High Intensity Focused Ultrasound is just High Intensity UltraSoundapplied through 10 cm long 2 cm thick guide tube. It has no benefit over HIUS. Actually less effective than High Intensity UltraSound.

Every couple of years they need to change the ultrasound device name to sell more ultrasound units. High Intensity Focused Ultrasoundhas no medical benefit. It is over specific.

So I applied HIUS for 10 seconds to my friends pancreas. Located at the bottom left of the rib cage.

I thought it might help reduce the severity of the diabetes. He was over keen when I next met him.

The medics at Salford Royal Hospital have found his pancreas has started excreting insulin again. After five years of total insulin dependent.

Medics always insisted that diabetes was caused by the destruction of insane stem cells. The beta cells.

It would take two weeks to repopulate the pancreas the new stem cells.

But the diabetes abated in 10 minutes. And there medics confirmed that his pancreas was making insulin again.

So the pathogen was being more circuitous. The viral rump helium produced by antisense enzyme to insulin. To block is biological function.

Or it may be inappropriate enzymes to deactivate the function of the stem cells. Hacking into the buyer regulation system of insulin production.

We don't need to know which. In the viral rump was overinflated-as shown by low power ultrasound scans.

So at 8 W the rump structure was converting ultrasound into X-ray radiation and dangerous levels of heat.

It also would have produced a tiny amount of helium and oxygen gases: as it did molecular nuclear fusion.

With HIUS the energy production by a viral rump is sufficient to cause cell content boiling.

Only happens in body cells above 180 W/cm2. So I only used fuel and licensed HIUS at 150 W 40 kHz. Now 8W 1MHz.

I used to work in ultrasound! Ironically my old boss retired and died of pancreatic cancer six months later.

During his working life the metallurgical ultrasound have protected Ian from cancer, diabetes and heart disease.

1 10 second application of HIUS gave for a faltering recovery from his diabetes!

He would have three days total remission from diabetes, then the any supplemental insulin for two. Than three days' remission again.

So the next time I saw him I got serious! I only had a cheap HIUS device because I had no idea it would actually work were bought it from China.

I gave him a 30 sections to his pancreas. Ten seconds to each armpit(I know not why). And 20 seconds to his brain and liver.

This time I have produced a total permanent remission from type two diabetes.

The next week he brought along a friend with type one diabetes. I HIUSed her, and never saw her again. So I presume she got a total remission. Maybe 3 day delay in acting. She needed 1 minute of High Intensity UltraSound.

I was in contact with America with type one diabetes. After two weeks discussion you apply the HIUS to his pancreas.

Again I never heard from him again! I charged him to apply the HIUS to always friends with diabetes.

I thought all this out on the Internet. They reckon good ideas travel around the world in four days.

I had emails about ultrasound and cancer. So as we talk the world is being cured of cancer. All so, so easy.

No biochemistry involved. By the time you read this my diabetes idea has also circle the world twice.

The HIUS device is fantastically cheap! An application of the ultrasound does not interfere with any fatal biochemical treatment you are subjected to.

At your next GP appointment they should find you are cancer or diabetes in remission.

The High Intensity UltraSound idea has been medically published by applying the ultrasound to the coronary arteries and the kidneys external to the body.

It clears the troublesome pathogen rump: again these are overinflated and hard! And lacking support from the dendrite mesh.

A lower power ultrasound scan will show remission from all the diseases of age.

The hardened white cells have vanished! Cancer is the simplest disease to fix.

Heart disease nearly as simple! As the pathogen rump is very prevalent.

With diabetes the pathogen rump is not as numerous. So we need to destroy all the diabetes causing cells with the ultrasound.

In cancer the immune system gets involved, to ensure the cancer cell type is cleared.

Aged people produce misty ultrasounds! As pathogen rumps accumulate through the body.

They may not be biologically active. They just have reduced the vitality of the whole body.

Or there may be growing fast like cancer. Or have dramatic actions on the body is Bio chemistry-as in diabetes.

The application of HIUS to the pancreas costs 5¢. It interferes with no biochemical treatment.

As mentioned above the GP should desist all biochemical prescriptions have at the next doctor's appointment.

High Intensity UltraSound was proved by the Moffitt in 2002. But this news was hidden by the drug companies!

By application of their money to suppress news of this exciting medical department in the world newspapers.

30 million people die every year as a result of cancer and the other diseases of age. Eight million people die from diabetes. 12 from heart disease.

All these diseases are totally fixable at one appointment using HIUS. Or if you prefer our HIFU-again no medical benefit in the new name.

So the drug companies have succeeded in killing a third of a billion people. Including our friends and family.

This is my informed opinion. I am waiting for my first objection to this idea from around the world.

Biochemical treatments produce expensive, unpleasant inevitable death.

Ultrasound produces a one appointment cure. For 5¢. The drug companies turn out to be the biggest mass killers in history.

A HIUS device is available over the Internet for 13 UK pounds, on E bay '8W 1MHGz ultrasound massage device cheapest'. It can be used to cure the diseases of age from minimum of 5000 people.

Then we need to track the cure to cancer, heart disease, high blood pressure, Diabetes-the diseases of age.

The devices are sold to clear scarring, and wrinkles, and the key motion of weight in old age.

I have first-hand experience of HIUS curing diabetes. Type one and type two.

At one application. No biochemistry involved.

Just as the Moffitt found which cancer!

Head injuries

I have a personal interest here. As discussed below HIFU can be used to clear cessated cells. Damaged cells in the CNS have available telomere. So they are not routinely cleared. Even when inactive.

Inactive cells contract, but still had taken cell room. A buzz of HIFU will cause such cells to rupture there cell walls. Then the macrophages will clear them.

This is important purpose final and head injuries. This is an area that needs more research. With an aged population head and spinal injuries are of growing importance.

Both traumatic injuries and infections can cause damage to the CNS. It is not an insoluble problem!. That is what I think-go and find out!

Mental illness

This is them a speculative area we could apply HIFU to. I have no personal knowledge of mental illness. I have returned his a high level psychiatric nurse, and he warns me not to get involved in this discipline. Which is horrendously complicated. But here goes.

Since my first degree I have been aware that there is a significant body of medical opinion that links mental illness to a chemical imbalance of the brain. This strikes me as classic pathogen leader activity.

I do know that infections turned to colonise the central nervous system as well as the lungs. The immune system has limited access to the CNS. The lungs give the pathogen easy distribution to the population.

After the infection is cleared throughout the body the diseases of age are caused by pathogen leaders warming bacterial or viral rumps. A part pathogen, that just affects the homoeostasis of the body.

Pathology which show if this idea is accurate! Dissecting the brains of individuals who had died with mental illness will show hard and pathogen leaders throughout the brain. Looking very reminiscent of slow growing cancer tumours.

All rump infestations are inflated to gain extra vitality-or they would coals no disease. This makes them especially susceptible to HIFU.

As ever ultrasound at 150 W 40 kHz will clear the troublesome rumps. I haven't mentioned above why 40 kilohertz. Ultrasonic carpet cleaners boil off water sprayed on the carpet. This is the same process that you want to induce in viral rumps to cause their fragmentation.

350 kilohertz is more effective. But I feel may be two had caustic in the body. We are inducing an immune action, so providing we cause significant cell damage, we are not to bothered we do not create complete cell clearance. The immune system will finish the job!

I mentioned this is a very speculative idea. My proof reader will be very leery of me being interested in this area of medicine. The GP surgery will have a HIFU unit at hand to cure cancer.

It will do no harm applying it to the brain. But many cure mental health problems from schizophrenia to other psychopathies. It will also clear depression and minor mental problems.

I am aware that manic depressives write excellent comedy. I write comedy, but I am aware that it partially de-hinges even a totally sane me! That's why he I don't write too much of it. I value my sanity too much.

Give them a but I can write comedy when feeling very balanced, I have no doubt that zany comedians would still do good work, and benefit from the use of my HIFU unit.

That is why I am concentrating on my singing and video making. That does not remotely affect my sanity level.

I am aware that PM T does cause some ladies to cure their partner! I would include PM T with other mental illnesses. Don't shout at me ladies. It just means regular use of the GP surgery HIFU machine may have worsened the mood swings induced.

Girls will protest that it is a hormone imbalance. Not all ladies have PM T. I think a pathogen leader in the CNS is a exacerbating the mood swings.

I would group it together with mental illness, as a neurological problem by HIFU. More than any other diseases of age people paid acknowledging mental illness.

Talking to Frank Bruno! Particularly if you are not white mental illness may be developed with age.

This is not racist! No more than the same light boxes, runners and athletes wipe the floor with white ones. As the world population ages this is granted are more and more important.

A quick buzz of HIFU will sort such problems out. Not acknowledging the wrong does not make it go away. Mental dullness is a severe problem for all racial groupings. Now we can fix it!

Slowing down the speed of ageing

This is the holy grail of medicine. Body cells are designed to have 50 lives, their be cleared and replaced from the stem cells. Even your bones are at the time by the immune system every 10 years. The rest of your body every four!

Viruses found an advantage in turning up biological activity in the cell so making the cell cessate with available telomere. The cell ceases is to be biologically active.

And just exists to copy the viral genome. Regular famines are no longer a factor of life. So we would rather cells with no telomere and viral altered cells were cleared.

Viruses are over excrete endothelial growth factor. This demands and gets extra blood supplies. So the cell is inflated and hard!

Cessated cells contract, and cease to be flaccid. So they are now compact and hard. This is our opportunity!

Applying HIFU routinely will clear such cells from the body. We are then left with the diseases experience in middle age. The diseases of age cease to be.

How we will age, I do not know. It will be down to copying errors from the stem cells. I'm convinced that all press and infectious disease can be cured by a buzz of ultrasound to the chest and head.

The HIFU device could be one of the most useful additions to the GP surgery. It will not make you last forever! Immortality was never going to be that easy.

Nature is even more inventive than man is. There are whole new classes of diseases out there waiting to kill us.

It is largely up to the geniuses at the NI H, Harvard and Cambridge universities to cope with the future.

It is a good job they have brains. They are going to need them!

A1 the medical cures

My friends are fortunate individuals. As I am gradually getting them all cures of the various conditions.

I had two non blood relatives who died of diabetes over 15 years ago. At the time I worked in medical ultrasound! But had no idea that it would help them.

A contact from America we diabetes has contacted me, as a result of my videos on diabetes on YouTube, to say it that HIFU does cure diabetes.

He did not say type 1 or 2. Does not matter! Both are caused by a viral rump in the pancreas-left behind from infective disease.

HIFU clears it at one application.

I have referred often to the work done in Florida Air in 2002 on prostate cancer. Prostate surgery has deficient therapeutic outcome.

Chemo and radio therapy are delayed unpleasant death! One application of ultrasound will clear the viral rump causing the cancer.

I do not have any friends with breast cancer! If you do, one application of ultrasound at 150 Watts 40 kHz will clear the most aggressive cancers out there.

The drug companies are trying to make out that HIFU has limited application. No it doesn't! It will cure all 200 sorts of cancer out there today.

Any new cancer will share the pressurised cancer cell nature that makes the cancer especially susceptible to HIFU. At power densities benign to body cells.

The bystander cell damage the destruction of the cancer cells creates, so there is an immune action to clear cancer throughout the body.

Probably have the single most important development I will be remembered for, is curing coronary heart disease. Not treating it! Curing it at one application.

I use three applications-as I am conservative! And the ultrasound does no damage to body cells. My proof reader has coronary heart disease.

He has no requested a copy of this book. So he can have a number and signed edition. So he can say that his friend wrote this book and cure coronary heart disease.

I am not a medical expert! Here are some medics tried out my idea on the coronary arteries. Which is actually inspired by some other medics who did pathology on coronary heart disease victims.

There may be a bacterial rump on the coronary arteries-that is what the pathology suggested! The medics tried out HIFU on the kidneys.

They have a major role in controlling blood pressure! They secrete the Rennin enzyme which controls the blood pressure created by the heart.

The bacterial rump inappropriately secretes this enzyme. So we end up with abnormally high and inappropriate blood pressure.

Application of high HIFU to kidneys has a 100% clearance rate for secondary coronary heart disease. Application of the ultrasound to the coronary arteries will clear the primary coronary heart disease.

My cleaner had arthritis in his right hand: as he is plunging his hands into water all day! So arthritis is probably an occupational hazards of that job.

Now we get personal! I have applied HIFU to my skull to fix by a pre-existing head injury. I suffered 30% brain damage in 1988.

I have extensive eye surgery to correct for A dormant natural abducting muscle in my eye.

My eyes are slightly misaligned vertically, but they now align horizontally. So lateral abductor muscle now works.

My proof reader said the ultrasound gave him a slight headache. This might occur on the first application. It is clearing defective cells from the brain. Future applications will not give the patient a headache.

I used to have thick hair. Now as I age my hair became less thick. Application of the ultrasound to sort out my head injury fake and my hair yet again!

February 2013 it appears that high intensity ultrasound could change human ageing totally. Curing both cancer and heart disease.

The ultrasound causes cell content boiling in the pressurised cancer cells. I was working on ultrasound producing nuclear fusion from regular water.

This is the system that cures cancer! Regular body cells are not pressurised and so I heated by 2° C while the cancer cell is heated past 60° C-at which the cancer is dead.

At 120° C the cancer cell fragments explosively. HIFU is the first course the medical treatment that does not damage body cells. That these to a one appointment cure of all cancers out there.

Today 12 million people die around the glow from coronary heart disease. HIFU cures this disease at one appointment.

8 million people will no longer die as a result of diabetes.